Cleuber Cristiano de Sousa

# Psychomotricity in Autistic Spectrum Disorder

Cleuber Cristiano de Sousa

# Psychomotricity in Autistic Spectrum Disorder

## The cognitive, the emotional and the motor

ScienciaScripts

# PSYCHOMOTRICITY IN AUTISTIC/AUTISM SPECTRUM DISORDER

The cognitive, the emotional and the motor.

Cleuber Cristiano de Sousa
Psychomotricist

# TABLE OF CONTENTS

# PRESENTATION

Motor and psychomotor activities are essential components for success in orchestrating the Sequential Plan of Action - PSA/Curriculum in the ability to play, social and motor, in the methodology of intervention in Autism Spectrum Disorder (TEA). When it is a physical activity that arouses orality (commands or echoes or tact) it is still a secondary positive enhancer (activity) in the performance of the most effective intervention based on the scientific studies of Applied Behavior Analysis - ABA. The result of this type of activity can be explained by means of compression of muscles and joints, as well as respiratory rate and heartbeat, while stressing the release of the action hormone (adrenaline and noradrenaline), preparing the body for effort and struggle or escape. The sensation of self-pleasure discharge can function as a mode of sensory *input*. An intervention of potential motor quality is the use of circuits, initially being a single circuit, and later, making the circuit mixed, for the articulation of fine and thick praxia, with levels of complexity. Thus, Psychomotricity, by relating the cognitive, the emotional and the motor, is indispensable for the development of abilities of children, adults and the elderly in Autistic Spectrum Disorder (299.00/F84.0).

The orthodoxy of positivist and strictly behavioural studies has imposed a duality between the autarchic body and mind that is measurable in the psychic and somato poles. Psychomotricity arises from the relationships between psychic and motor activities, of a transdisciplinary nature, extrapolating their activities to the construction of possible realities to be reached, in order to accommodate biological and mental processes.

By relating the field of emotions (limbic system) and the affectivity of a symbolic universe to the five neurological motor subsystems (pyramidal, extrapyramidal, medullar, reticular and cerebellar), the symbolic representations and ideas relate inseparably to motor activities, which are no longer understood as the materialization of the psychism.

The orientation of an integrality of a subject immersed in self-knowledge and self-evaluation involved with the maximization of social relationships and committed to the objects of his psyche allows the transversalization of the biological, physiological and psychic to be immanent to the body as the mediation of being.

Thus, in the studies of psychomotricity, the human motor act is integrated into the social mediation relations of the subject in his psychic reality. In this work, efforts are made to present this relational reality, contributing to the achievement of positive results with regard to interventions in psychomotricity both in institutions and clinics.

Psychomotor development is linked to the maturation of the organism, and the cognitive components (cognition), biological functions and affectivity have as their genesis the body.

For an analysis of the functioning and integration of the systems that are in the entangled psychomotor development it is necessary to understand the relationships between stimulation, integration and response system. Each system has very specific functions at very significant stages of evolution.

The stimulation system is in charge of receiving external and internal information from the organs responsible for sensations and passing on the messages to the integration system, which is responsible for the process and subsequent storage of the information that will contribute to activate the planning, memory and consciousness and other components of perception, with the role of the response system being to externalize the information and messages processed and made operational by the motor action.

The principles of human development are given in stages with specific characteristics that define in a particular way the periodization of the evolution of the being. For Gesell (1998),

*the cycle of human development is continuous. All growth is based on previous growth. The development process is thus a paradoxical mix of creation and perpetuation. (p. 27).*

The verticality in the systematization of the seven factors that contribute to the global organization of psychomotricity refers to the tonicity occurring by means of neuromuscular acquisition and integration of antigravidic motor patterns. The period of perception of these elements is between birth and 12 months of age of the child. They are of three types: support, rest and posture.

The balance appears between the 12 months of the child and the 2 years of age offer security and the evolution of the patterns of locomotion, both manifested in the acquisition of bipedal posture. The laterality appears from 2 to 3 years, through the afferent systems, diffuse perceptions, emotional investment and sensory integration.

Body awareness, imitation behaviours and their respective perception appear from 3 to 4 years of age developed through the body scheme and image. It is in the awareness of one's own body and of attitudes and posture that the development of the body scheme is conceived. The mental representation of the body by the subject is what is called body image.

Language proficiency and spatial and temporal coordination appear between 4 and 5 years and manifest themselves through selective attention being called spatial temporal structuring in the body domain. It is in the integral perception of global praxis and occurring through the hand-eye and foot-eye coordination, inclusion of rhythm and planning of all motor coordination that the perception appears between 5 and 6 years. The fine praxia, between 6 and 7 years, occurs in the hemispheric specialization, through concentration and its respective organization.

The development of psychomotor activities and methodologies as a playful skill is immersed in the universe of the Psychomotricist's making.

In this work, three academic skills of relational psychomotricity will be presented: motor skills, play and language.

The measurability markers will be: duration, frequency and intensity and the inputs may be materials adapted to the activity.

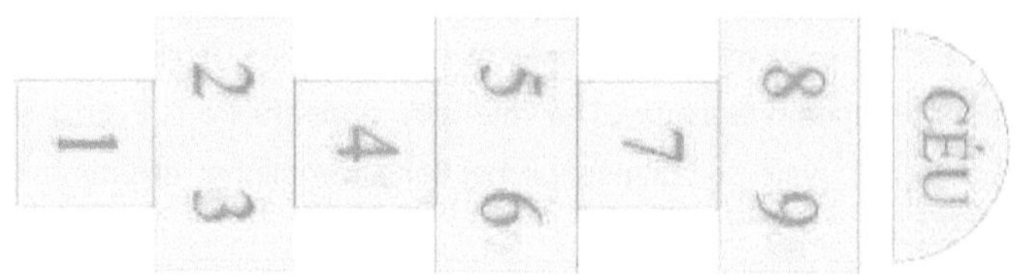


Fig 1. School of Health in Psychosomatic Medicine - ESMP/2020

| Item | Activity | Skill | Frequency | Intensity | Duration |
|---|---|---|---|---|---|
| 1 | Amarelinha | Play | Indefinite | Take it to | Indefinite |
| 2 | Amarelinha | Engine | 2 | Moderated | 30 min |
| 3 | Amarelinha | Communication | 2 | Take it to | 30 min |
| Inputs | Chalk for drawing, weight and notepad. | | | | |
| Age | 5 to 7 years | | | | |
| HP[1] | Thin Motor Balance/Coordination and Body Schematic | | | | |
| Description | Activity in which the subject jumps over a layout/drawing that does not follow a linear geometric shape. The play/play begins with the child throwing the weight (rectangular object) into the space of the listed region (1). Afterwards, it jumps on one foot (balance) in the other houses/regions until it reaches a circular space called sky, respecting the lines. When arriving at the "sky" it jumps with two feet. The geometry will offer through the lines the spatiality and laterality, as well as the application. The development of the ability to use small muscles in pierced and detailed movements: drawing, writing, disassembling, unbuttoning and buttoning (tying and untied). | | | | |

**[1] developed/psychomotor skills**
**Fig 2. School of Health in Psychosomatic Medicine - ESMP/2020**

Psychomotricity is responsible for investigating the changes in the relationship between the individual and his social universe and the relationships with his social brain. This space of movement is made up of cognitive, emotional, affective, cultural elements, etc. Interdisciplinarity is responsible for the dialogue between the objects of study of the most diverse disciplines and the study of psychomotor development is closely related to the most diverse areas of knowledge, with great contributive value. The proximity and articulation between psychomotricity and disciplines such as Philosophy, Biology and the like have such a connection and crossing that borders, limits and domains become impossible to demarcate.

Play (yellow) in the context of Psychomotricity needs in its field of investigation studies and research that enable the understanding of the factors inherent in the teaching and learning processes, as well as the understanding of the elements that surround the subject and enable his positioning as a being in the world and his social relations with the other (body, mind and social relationships), from the perspective of neuropsychomotor and cognitive components: memory, attention, thought, perception, problem solving and reasoning.

Thus, studies that also combine Developmental Psychology, Learning Psychology and Psychology in Education come together in studies of great value to the intra- and extra-school context of Psychomotricity. Vygotsky's developmental studies have their reference in the active construction, in the relationships established with the social environment, the environment that proposes itself as a mediator of this individual in his singularity and the relationship with his peers. Vygostsky (1978) institutes that in order to study children's development, one must begin with a dialectical understanding between two radically different lines: the biological and the cultural. To adequately study such a process, it is necessary to know these two components and the laws which govern their interplay at each stage of children's development.

The formation of motor and mental operations responsible for comparison, division, order, quantification, applicability, prehension is essential for the appropriation of human characteristics. The interaction between the individual and the social world is capable of accelerating or delaying the formation of these abilities, and the lack of stimulus (social behaviorism) impairs the physical and biological reactions that incorporate this cognitive construct. The more access one has to objects and materials, the greater the possibilities of associations and, thus, the experiential experiences will result in the appropriation of the meanings and resignified of these objects and situations.

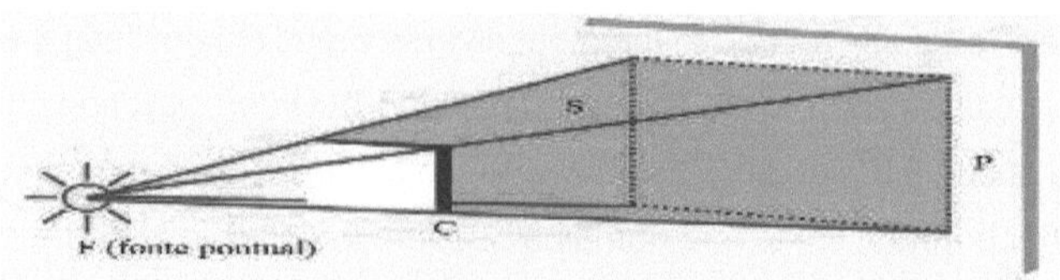

Fig 3. School of Health in Psychosomatic Medicine - ESMP/2020

| Item | Shadow | Penumbra | Light |
|------|--------|----------|-------|
| 1 | Meanings | Re-designated | Objects |

**School of Health in Psychosomatic Medicine - ESMP/2020**

Psychomotricity in educational, institutional and clinical contexts as a process of dialectic and dialogical analysis is based on social practice. The study of the phases of development, of learning and of the school environment enables a vertical and not only horizontal understanding of the imbricated relationships of this do that besides being motor, is psychic, in an inseparable relationship. The conceptions of man and his relationship with the social environment contribute to the understanding of the constitution of the subject placed in relation to the social and symbolic.

The multiple intelligences as a whole favour a mapping of their stimuli and motivation, of this awareness that the body is no longer seen as externalizing the psyche. The Psychomotricist in possession of these theoretical-methodological devices can organize and plan activities in diverse environments (internal and external) that will promote the interpretation of social reality based on concrete everyday situations.

Psychomotricity is a process that operates knowledge essential for overcoming difficulties and developing learning, with regard to losses in cognitive, motor, psychic and social components.

The clinic in the context of psychomotricity is a constitutive process of man's social and cultural identity. Mental operations and social behaviour are related so that formal schooling can be the transforming instrument of emancipation from being in situations of overcoming.

The conceptions of development, with their theoretical currents and repercussions on the school, signal the assumptions for the role of interactions of internal and external factors. The inatist, environmentalist, and interactionist conceptions propose an understanding of whether or not the subject is distant from his or her research object proposed by the researcher, who is a teacher. Psychomotricity theories relate, transversalize, articulate, and enable the necessary intervention in the clinic and institution.

On this subject, then, it can be said that school is not the appropriate space for the identification, classification or diagnosis of a child who presents signs and symptoms of an autistic disorder. But it must be stressed that the fact that the teacher is not prepared for this work does not rule out the significant number of children in autism (light and moderate) in school units.

The presentation of problems of alternative social or emotional interaction, serious problems to maintain relationships or develop social engagement activities, as well as presenting difficulties of nonverbal communication, thus including gestural, vocal, postural, abnormality in eye movements and facial expressions and the non-recognition of facial expressions as signs in other people are symptoms attributed to Autism/TEA/Autism Spectrum Disorder.

Life in society allows the apprehension and planning, direction and evaluation of your action. This process of identity building, which is organised and self-organised by cultural limits and its boundaries, mistakes are essential for reflection on it and, in the meantime, adjustment of conduct is possible.

Correction" is an important factor for understanding, storage and reproduction, but in TEA/Autism this action is done by exhaustive and sequential repetition, in order to reinforce desirable behaviors and replace those that are undesirable. When the desire to integrate is manifested, otherness is perceived as a basic need for the insertion of man in a social environment. It is from this reference that the Applied Behavioural Analysis acts, by means of methodologies, academic skills (social, motor, play, personal and language) in a PSA/ curriculum adapted and centred on motivation and reward, by means of positive reinforcers.

The clinical activities carried out by simulation of the social environment provide the necessary variables for the formation of identity and the operationalization of consciousness, which is already formed. This consciousness corresponds to the nature capable of discerning between the objective and material questions belonging to the individual's social reality and the subjective elements of the context of life. The work is responsible for the organization of many elements and experiential factors that provoke paradoxes, contradictions and coincidences, contributing to the social counterpoints of dialectical category.

Psychomotricity is responsible for investigating the changes in the relationship between the individual and his social universe and the relationships with his social brain. This space of movement is made up of cognitive, emotional, affective, cultural elements, etc. Interdisciplinarity is responsible for the dialogue between the objects of study of the most diverse disciplines and psychology is closely related to the most diverse areas of knowledge, with great contributive value. The closeness and articulation between psychology and disciplines such as Philosophy, Biology and the like have such a connection and crossing that borders, limits and domains become impossible to demarcate.

Vygotsky has the reference in the active construction, in the relations established with the social environment, environment that proposes itself as mediator of this individual in his singularity and the relationship with his peers. Vygotsky (1978) also institutes that in order to study children's development, one must begin with a dialectical understanding between two radically different lines: the biological and the cultural. To adequately study such a process, it is necessary to know these two components and the laws which govern their interplay at each stage of children's development.

The formation of motor and mental operations responsible for comparison, division, order, quantification, applicability, prehension is essential for the appropriation of human characteristics. The interaction between the individual and the social world is capable of accelerating or delaying the formation of these abilities, and the lack of stimulus (social behaviorism) impairs the physical and biological reactions that incorporate this cognitive construct. The more access one has to objects and materials, the greater the possibilities of associations and, thus, the experiential experiences will result in the appropriation of the meanings and resignified of these objects and situations.

The perceptual and motor evolution of intellectual functions, sociability and the affectivity of the human being, is the object of analysis of human development and it is through this that the description of how these capacities evolve and how this occurs and what implication this has on the social response of the individual in his most diverse daily situations is proposed.

Leontiev opposes biological opinions on the nature and development of the human psyche. Leontiev states that in order to learn concepts, generalizations, knowledge, the child must form appropriate mental actions. This presupposes that these actions are actively organized. Initially, they take the form of external actions which adults form in the child and only then do they become internal mental actions.

The active appropriation of man's social experience is what is called learning. The interactions and horizons of expectations that are broadened in the course of experiential experiences are responsible for the network of meanings and resignifications.

Thus, learning studies aim at the analysis of the complexity in the process by which the multiple ways of having an impression, of understanding, of thinking and the various types of knowledge (philosophical, theological, empirical) are apprehended in society and appropriated by the social agent. Knowledge and recognition of the social nature of learning is a *sine qua non* factor for understanding this process. Social mediations are responsible for the formation of cognitive operations, which are in the process of the action of knowing.

In the Psychomotricity Clinic, the child's social relationships are maximised with regard to difficulties, disorders and learning disorders, and then a significant transformation is perceived in the way the child thinks, conceives reality, processes messages and performs the formal operations already conceived. Psycho-pedagogical knowledge contributes to the extent that it enables more precise clinical planning even if in the classroom as an open system there are interventions and from them the initial conditions for self-organisation are resumed. The clinic is a space that favors the understanding of the mental and social processes of the agent in action in a non-linear, non deterministic and non-mechanistic world.

The developmental terms are based on different conceptions of man and his relationship with the social environment. The explanation of reality is the result of the world view and the historical, cultural and social determination of a specific moment. The inactist conception is based on spontaneous development and the environment must interfere sensitively in this process. Values, beliefs, habits, the way they think, their social conduct and their emotional reactions are inherent to man. The origin comes from a theological position and is also related to Darwin's evolutionist proposal, embryology and genetics.

The PSA/Curriculum should ensure psychomotricity (balance, laterality, spatiality, location, gravity and application). Daily actions (running, jumping and stretching) are rearranged as a goal of self-regulation, calmness, balancing and modulation of the respiratory rate, replacing repetitive and ritualistic actions with reorganization actions, search for physical sensations by multimodality. If the child is presented with a yellowish circuit, besides balancing and spatiality for quadrant adjustment, the brain will be focused on the development of activity by precision, that is, disruptive behaviors will be minimized.

# INDIVIDUAL PSYCHOMOTOR COUNSELLING FORM

<table>
<tr><td colspan="2" align="center">Concepts</td></tr>
</table>

| SEQ | MOTOR COOORDINATION SKILLS |
|---|---|
| 01 | You have mastery of your body image; |
| 02 | Elaborates alternate movements; |
| 03 | Elaborates synchronized movements; |
| 04 | It develops complementary lower limb movements; |
| 05 | It develops complementary movements of upper limbs; |
| 06 | It presents acquisition of lateral movements (lateral notion); |
| 07 | It has a perception of spatiality (spatial notion); |
| 08 | It articulates spatiality (spatial notion), laterality (lateral notion) and temporality (temporal notion); |
| 09 | It presents body scheme efficiency; |
| 10 | It has control of global motor coordination (broad musculature in complex movements); |
| 11 | Uses fine motor coordination in an appropriate and dynamic way (small muscles). |
| Total | |
| SEQ | SKILLS IN THE AREA OF SOCIABILITY |
| 12 | It analyses and interprets and formulates social situations of interaction and reciprocity; |
| 13 | It uses different methods to interact and relate in known and unknown environments; |
| 14 | It presents impaired social responses; |
| 15 | It has balance and keeps calm in changing situations; |
| 16 | Understands and interprets situations involving social issues of interest to you; |
| 17 | It interprets and understands situations involving social issues that are not of common interest to it; |
| 18 | It presents fixation on themes of its interest; |
| 19 | It is easy to change patterns of interest; |
| 20 | It organizes and participates in group activities; |
| 21 | It presents a normal social approach; |
| 22 | Has participation and interest in joining a group or participating in social activities. |
| Total | |
| SEQ | SKILLS IN THE AREA OF AFFECTIVITY |
| 23 | It uses strategies to relate and show affection; |
| 24 | It uses different procedures to externalize general feelings; |
| 25 | It expresses particular feelings (family, friends and personal); |
| 26 | It values receiving compliments or showing affection; |

| SEQ | |
|---|---|
| 27 | Understands and interprets situations involving affective and social issues; |
| 28 | It develops the affectivity of different methods (social media, letters, music, videos and other genres); |
| 29 | It socially demonstrates its affective intentions (expresses the feeling in public); |
| 30 | It presents self-knowledge and self-assessment (self-affectiveness); |
| 31 | Organizing events, activities or social interactions that consolidate affectivity; |
| 32 | It is easy to share themes of expression of your emotions and affection. |
| 33 | He participates and is interested in collective celebrations and experiences the group's achievements. |
| Total | |
| **SEQ** | **PLAYING SKILLS** |
| 34 | It presents balance during playful and playful activities; |
| 35 | It uses different procedures to achieve the objectives demonstrating strength and agility; |
| 36 | It demonstrates organisation and expresses results, building leadership; |
| 37 | It characterises and values issues of environmental balance and conservation; |
| 38 | Understands and interprets situations involving health, biological, affective and social issues; |
| 39 | It presents anxiety control, using systematization and segmentation (steps/steps); |
| 40 | Elaboration, exercise and demonstration of symbols, imagination and fantasy; |
| 41 | It demonstrates mutual respect and good sociability with its peers and social groups; |
| 42 | It presents articulation, organization, systematization and cooperation, with an exercise of solidarity; |
| 43 | It develops activities that demonstrate motor coordination skills (global and fine); |
| 44 | He participates and is interested in playful activities, demonstrating his ability to memorize. |
| Total | |
| **SEQ** | **PERSONAL CARE SKILLS** |
| 45 | It presents autonomy in personal hygiene (bath); |
| 46 | It presents autonomy in personal hygiene (oral); |
| 47 | Organises your activities and makes use of your personal care skills in part; |
| 48 | It characterises and values issues of cooperation and body care and hygiene; |
| 49 | Understands and interprets situations involving personal health; |
| 50 | It has an articulated notion of spatiality, laterality and temporality; |
| 51 | Autonomy is perceived when using the bath (physiological needs); |

| 52 | It presents hydration awareness, corresponding to the act of drinking water when one is thirsty; |
|---|---|
| 53 | It uses personal belongings in an organised and systematic way; |
| 54 | It needs cooperation and help in the use of personal belongings; |
| 55 | Self-evaluates and recognises the relationship between image and hygiene in personal care. |
| Total | |
| **SEQ SEQ** | **COMMUNICATION AND LANGUAGE SKILLS** |
| 56 | Make a habit of reading verbally, nonverbally and paraverbally with fluency; |
| 57 | It has good diction and intonation. It writes coherent, cohesive and creative texts; |
| 58 | It has good writing and makes use of grammar (correct spelling); |
| 59 | It uses mechanisms of meaning and textual use relations (comparison, substitution, gradation, etc.); |
| 60 | Use of contextualization and prior knowledge; |
| 61 | He makes use of dictionary terms and understands the analogies and how to use them; |
| 62 | The use of foreignisms and their contextualised use; |
| 63 | It translates and forms sense relationships, comes as language loans; |
| 64 | It expresses ideas, expressions, feelings and plasticity in the relationships between text and cotext; |
| 65 | It makes use of images and relations of verbal, non-verbal and paraverbal texts; |
| 66 | It makes use of expressionism and artistic and imagetic forms; |
| 67 | It takes care of the formatting and relations of form and content of the texts; |
| 68 | It proposes and participates in the production of individual and collective texts and art; |
| 69 | He has acuity, proselytism, punctuality and assiduity in his productions and artistic activities; |
| 70 | It socialises and respects the artistic and cultural diversity of productions and linguistic and textual diversity; |
| 71 | It performs critical analysis and interprets language relationships; |
| 72 | It systematises, organises and relates to linguistic, textual and cultural diversity; |
| 73 | It proposes interdisciplinary and transdisciplinary activities. |
| Total | |
| **SEQ** | **SKILLS IN THE HUMANITIES AREA** |
| 74 | It has information spatial and temporal orientation; |
| 75 | It uses techniques and technologies in different contexts of history and geography; |
| 76 | It carries out the interpretation and analysis of cartography and geographical location; |
| 77 | Has analysis and critical interpretation of texts and information |
| 78 | It orders and systematises dates, geographical location and political, social, philosophical and cultural aspects; |

| 79 | It has well-founded opinions and ideas on subjects of various kinds; |
|---|---|
| 80 | It undertakes critical analysis and positions itself on historical and social issues; |
| 81 | It comprises themes, theories and definitions of historical and social moments; |
| 82 | He is curious, researcher and investigative; |
| 83 | It knows how to respect cultural, religious and political diversity; |
| 84 | Serve the next one cordially; |
| 85 | It is solidary and empathetic in everyday situations; |
| 86 | It is attentive and cares and interacts in the most different situations; |
| 87 | He is willing to cooperate with the group and has a team spirit; |
| 88 | Presents itself to various types of activities even if it is not of particular interest |
| Total | |
| **SEQ** | **NATURAL SCIENCE AND MATHEMATICS SKILLS** |
| 89 | Solves complex problems in a simple way; |
| 90 | It uses differentiated methodologies to arrive at common results; |
| 91 | It makes use of dialectics (deconstruction and reconstruction) in a rational way; |
| 92 | It articulates standards of conservation and socio-environmental preservation; |
| 93 | Rationally, it relates universal issues of philosophy and sociology; |
| 94 | It acts in a sensitive way and logical issues that are not accessible to the group; |
| 95 | It is thoughtful and rationally logical; |
| 96 | It articulates its premises in the particular context of group discussions; |
| 96 | It is faithful to its ideals in a balanced and rational way; |
| 98 | It participates in multiple activities without losing its integrity and reason. |
| 99 | It allows logical insertions to themes of a symbolic nature; |
| 100 | It has logical responsiveness. |
| Total | |
| Counting | |

**School of Health in Psychosomatic Medicine - ESMP/2020**

The elaboration of a PSA/Curriculum HP/M - Psychomotricity/Movement allows orientation, spatiality, laterality and balance (fine and thick praxia). Besides this ability, the behavior that extends to the cognitive, emotional and motor, must be related to the operationalization of cognitive components. The language, memory, attention, thought, reasoning and problem solving. Attention is an indispensable component for carrying out activities that demand precision. By committing oneself to contemplate this requirement, there will be a decrease in repetitive and ritualistic actions.

The adapted activities should correspond to the proposal of the Applied Behavior Analysis - ABA activities, its Sequential Action Plan, Curriculum and methodologies, as well as skills that will be sequentially developed according to the planning, which should be elaborated with effective participation of the family. Disruptive behavior harms concentration and in very specific cases of stereotypes that are self-injury is still a risk to the child's physical integrity. The sports activities adapted and planned in the ABA activities propose a substitute behaviour for the circumscribed interests that demand stereotypes. Changes in shifts or activity segments of the developed circuit or even the proposed exercise must take into account the diagnostic criteria B2 and B3 (Insistence on Same and Fixed Interests/DSM 5 (2013), which insert restricted interests, abnormality and intensity and focus, as well as inflexible adherence and ritualized routines and patterns of verbal behaviour.

Modelling is then needed to overcome the proposed situations that would take the child out of the comfort zone, but which could lead to fear and irritability, through adherence and rigid thinking patterns. These emotions and feelings should be orchestrated by the applicator, before proposing the operationalization of the activity, planning the possible behaviours that would result from the anxiety, stress and irritability by this attachment to repetitive, circumscribed and persevering behaviours.

The Autistic Spectrum Disorder Behaviour Analysis has in its scope the orientation to insert methodologies (EI/CV/TRD/TTD) aiming at the diversification of the child's behavioral repertoire, through the development of academic, personal, social language and motor skills. The B4 diagnostic criteria for Autism Spectrum Disorder/TEA/Autism, by DSM 5 (2013), presents for hyper or hyperreactivity, sensory stimuli or unusual interest in sensory aspects and reaction contrary to sounds or textures. These behaviours are related to imprecision in the decoding of sensory stimuli. Functional evaluation can provide a safe route for planning sensory desensitization or integration in order to regulate the organism. Several activities with different stimuli can be presented and the faults and gaps of imprecision can be verified from contact, which should then be related to the activities with regard to both desensitization and sensory integration.

| Item | Textures | Sensory stimulation |
|---|---|---|
| 1 | Compression | Lycra, towel, hydrotherapy cap, waistcoat, compression shirt. |
| 2 | Aspersion | Sandpaper, sponge and polisher, rough texture of a wall or of a rope and sea shells. |
| 3 | Softness | Soft fabric, cotton, blanket, plush, doll's hair. |
| 4 | Luminosity | Light toys, lamps, chandeliers, lanterns, traffic lights. |
| 5 | Gelatines | Pasta, gelatine adhesives, gelatinous cube, slime. |
| 6 | Bristles | Brush, toothbrush, brush, feather, feather duster, carpet with bristles. |
| 7 | Proprioceptive | Elastic bed, inflatable proprioceptive disc, proprioceptive ball, ball pool, rice, beans, pasta. Activities involving position and application. Multimodality activities. |

**School of Health in Psychosomatic Medicine - ESMP/2020**

## PSYCHO-PEDAGOGICAL/PSYCHOPATHOLOGICAL DIAGNOSIS

The psycho-pedagogical diagnosis of Autistic Spectrum Disorder - TEA, the analysis is based on observation, explanation and association with the environment, behavior and learning, as a process of systematic articulation of the child's activities. The association has as parameters the criteria established in the Diagnostic and Statistical Manual of Mental Disorders - DSM 5 (APA, 2013).

The signs and symptoms of Autistic Spectrum Disorder - TEA should appear in the early years of life, compromising both their social, linguistic and motor skills. These abilities are related to their cognitive skills: language, thinking, perception, memory, reasoning. So, because it is a neurobiological disorder that compromises the prefrontal cortex, it is important to point out that this area is mature after approximately 25 years of age.

This child's ability to relate to the environment will be severely impaired and it is from this association between environment, human behaviour and learning that the intervention activities will be applied. It is important at this juncture to understand the scope of the spectrum name. There is an umbrella effect on the semantic constitution of this word, achieving by expanding the classification F.84 to F.84.9/CID 10 (Artmed, 2013).

It is important to observe the diagnostic criteria present in neurodevelopment disorders (299.00/F84.0) with deficits that are persistent in various contexts present in media and interaction, with motor damage.

| RECIPROCITY SOCIOEMOTIONAL | BEHAVIOUR COMMUNICATIVE | UNDERSTANDING OF RELATIONSHIPS |
| --- | --- | --- |
| Abnormal social approach | Damage to non-verbal communication | Deficit of adaptation to social contexts |
| Harmful social responses | Variation of verbal and non-verbal communication deficit poorly integrated with abnormality | Damage in sharing imaginary jokes |
| Reduced sharing of interests, emotions or affection | Deficit in understanding facial gestures and expressions | Disinterest in peers and enturmation |
| Diagnostic criteria A1 | A2 diagnostic criteria | A3 diagnostic criteria |

Source: Brazilian Association of Psychosomatic Medicine-MT/2020

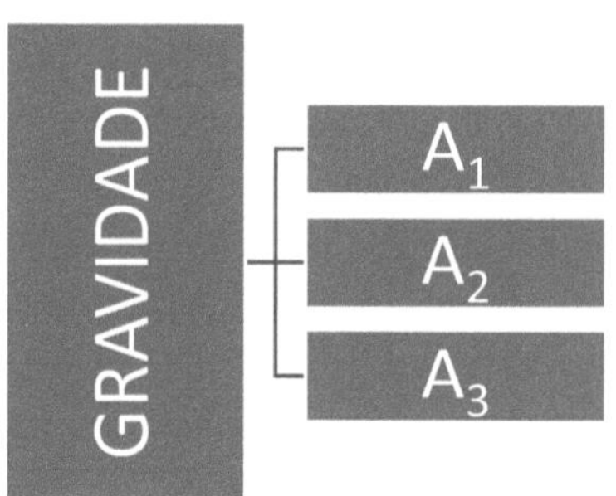


Source: Brazilian Association of Psychosomatic Medicine-MT/2020

| MOVEMENTS ENGINES | INSISTANCE IN MESMICE | INTERESTS FIXES | HIPER OR HYPORREATIVITY |
|---|---|---|---|
| Inappropriate use of objects | Unrelenting adherence to routines | Restricted interests | Sensory stimuli or unusual interest in sensory aspects |
| Stereotyped or repetitive speech, echolalia and idiosyncratic phrases | Ritualized patterns of verbal behaviour | Abnormality and intensity and focus | Apparent indifference to pain/temperature, reaction contrary to sounds or textures |
| Simple motor stereotype, aligning toys or rotating objects | Rigid standards of thought and eating the same food daily | Attachment to unusual objects, circumscribed or persevering interests | Visual fascination by light or movement |
| Criteria diagnostics B1 | Criteria B2 diagnostics | Criteria B3 diagnostics | Criteria B4 diagnostics |

Source: Brazilian Association of Psvchosomatic Medicine-MT/2020

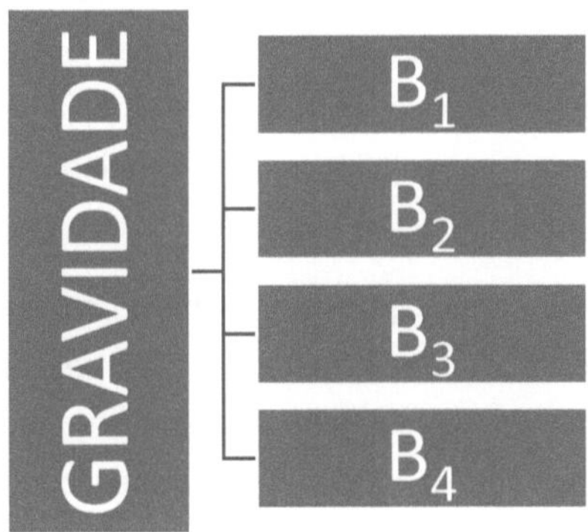


Source: Brazilian Association of Psychosomatic Medicine-MT/2020

The word "spectrum" indicates that when we speak of the autism disorder, we mean that there are different degrees or levels of this disorder for each child. In other words, children diagnosed with autism may present greater or lesser difficulties depending on the degree of the disorder manifested. DSM-5 provides for three levels of commitment (levels 1, 2 and 3). Level 1 is the level of least commitment and Level 3 is the level of most severe signs.

| Symptoms present early | Clinically significant damage to social and professional functioning. | Specify: with or without concomitant intellectual impairment, with or without concomitant language impairment, with catatonia. |
| --- | --- | --- |
| Diagnostic criteria C | Diagnostic criteria D | Diagnostic criteria E |



It is in etiopathogeny that the nosological diagnosis of Autism Spectrum Disorder is based, being a field of classification of disorders, of an explanatory nature. In Nosography, what is presented is a written exposition, a description of the diseases, with specific orientation to precise diagnosis and intervention/interventions for an effective treatment.

It is known that clinically the physiological alterations in language are not limited to the biological aspects of neurodevelopment, but it is from these limits that we will express our fundamental considerations about the relationship of the language/learning binomial. The damages in language acquisition and how it affects school development have multifactorial causes, but neurological factors are the reference for diagnosis and psycho-pedagogical interventions in treatment.

The importance of this study lies in the estimated prevalence of the TEA in 1% of the population, 70 million people in the world, 2 million of them in Brazil. In the

United States, a report from March 2014, the CDC - Center for Disease Control and Prevention, presented prevalence data of 1 in 54 boys with *Autism Spectrum Disorder. In 2016, in all 11 sites, the prevalence of TEA was 18.5 per 1,000 (one in 54) children aged 8 years and TEA was 4.3 times more prevalent among boys than girls. The prevalence of TEA varies according to location, ranging from 13.1 (Colorado) to 31.4 (New Jersey).*

*The prevalence estimates were approximately identical for non-Hispanic (white), non-Hispanic (black) and Asian / Pacific island children (18.5, 18.3 and 17.9, respectively), but lower for Hispanic children (15.4).*

*Among children with TEA for whom data on intellectual or cognitive functioning were available, 33% were classified as intellectually disabled (intelligence quotient [IQ] ≤70); this percentage was higher among girls than boys (39%versus 32%) and among black and Hispanic children than white (47%, 36% and 27%, respectively).*

*Black children with TEA were less likely to make a first assessment at 36 months than white children with TEA (40% versus 45%). The overall average age at the earliest known ASD diagnosis (51 months) was similar by sex and racial and ethnic groups; however, black children with IQ ≤70 had a later median age at ASD diagnosis than white children with IQ ≤70 (48 months versus 42 months). (Autism **Spectrum Disorder Prevalence in 8-Year-Old Children - Autism and Developmental Disabilities Monitoring Network, 11 Sites, United States, 2016 - Surveillance Abstracts / March 27, 2020/ Vol. 69 (4); 1-12- CDC - Centers for Disease Control and Prevention).***

Recent studies in Sweden in 2014 demonstrated a major sociocultural shift in estimates based on previous research. The authors are researchers at King's College, London, and the Karolinska Institute, Stockholm, and have stated that genetics has a weight of 50%, well below previous estimates of 80 to 90%, according to *JAMA, Journal of the American Medical Association.*

The UN - United Nations, in declaring April 2 - the World *Autism Awareness* Day, made possible a macro discussion that coincides with the objective of this research, which is the articulation between education, language and disorder of the autistic spectrum.

On this subject, then, it can be said that school is not the appropriate space for the identification, classification or diagnosis of a child who presents signs and symptoms of autistic disorder. But it must be stressed that the fact that the teacher is not prepared for this work does not rule out the significant number of children in a state of autism (light and moderate) in school units.

According to Portal Brasil, with information from the Ministry of Education, the Federal Government, in 2014 more than 698 thousand students, with special characteristics, were enrolled in common classes, with the percentage increasing 93%, in public schools.

Law 12.764, of 27 December 2012, discusses the National Policy for the Protection of the Rights of Persons with Autism Spectrum Disorders. The Ministry of Health's April 2013 Autism Spectrum Disorder Rehabilitation Care Guidelines (TEA) presents the guidelines to the Disability Care Network. There is still, as part of this legal framework, the Decree No. 8,368 of December 2, 2014, which regulates Law No. 12,764 of December 27, 2012, which establishes the National Policy for the Protection of the Rights of Persons with Autism Spectrum Disorders.

ICD 10 - International Statistical Classification of Diseases and Health Related Problems, in its tenth edition, has nine relational disorders in Global Development Disorders. As a reference, symptoms such as social aversion, difficulties in the development of the imagination, motor stereotypes, language with significant deviations are presented, these symptomatic manifestations being observed before the third year of childhood life.

About the ICD - International Statistical Classification of Diseases and Health Related Problems - ICD - 10, it is important to note that it is also called the International Classification of Diseases and unlike the DSM, it was published by WHO - World Health Organization and aims to present a standard in the formal use of disease codes.

The Diagnostic and Statistical Manual of Mental Disorders, in its fifth edition, DSM-5, significantly changed the diagnostic criteria for what was called autism. The presentation of symptoms early on and the impairment of the individual's ability to practice their activities in their daily lives are two references strongly highlighted by the new DSM review on Autism Spectrum Disorder.

In 1943, Leo Kanner presented for the first time the characteristics of ecolalia, obsessiveness, stereotyping and extreme autism for the term he described as Autistic Affective Contact Disorder. These writings already note a relationship with the intensity of imaginative life, alienism, and the absence of responses to stimuli from outside.

This term (autism) is a caudatory of Bleuler's studies, which, by means of AA/4A, presented that, for schizophrenia, the symptoms inherent in the orientation towards subjective life which alters the perception of the world (autism in Eugen Bleuler's conception), lack of unity of consciousness, presence of characteristic symptoms, evolution with inevitable deterioration and a multidimensional construction should be identified. What was called 4 A(s), by E. Bleuler, are 6 symptoms, ambivalence, blunted affection, associations and dissociations of thought, loss of attention, blunted affection, autism.

It is important to point out again that in DSM revision number 5, the subcategories of autism disorders are discarded, and the subcategories are grouped in a unified condition called Autism Spectrum Disorder - TEA. Asperger's Syndrome is not considered in a singular way, this condition being related to the global diagnosis of autism, which is now guided by two categories: presence of repetitive and stereotyped behaviour and alteration of the media.

The laws establishing the National Policy for the Protection of the Rights of Persons with Autism Spectrum Disorder are, first, Law No. 12.764 of 27 December 2012 and Decree No. 8.368 of 2 December 2014. In this Decree, the person with autistic spectrum disorder is considered a person with disability, for all legal purposes, this being a particularity of this disorder.

## TAB - ANALYSIS OF BEHAVIOUR APPLIED

Applied Behaviour Analysis is an area of knowledge that extends to the observation, analysis, explanation associated with the method, human behavior, learning and the environment, with regard to observality, monitoring, monitoring and controllability of management and guidance that, by relating to daily life and applying sequencing procedures to the daily life of the learner, has been well accepted and suggested for follow-up of children in Autism Spectrum Disorder, with reference to its spectrum, with likelihood of significant results in ICD(s) F.84.0 and F.84.1 (Child and atypical) from ICD 10.

This approach should be developed 1/1, with an applicator/teacher for each attended/learner, which besides having theoretical bases and scientific principles can be extended to other areas of knowledge, thus potentiating their capacity of interdisciplinarity and articulation for effective results in intervention and treatment. By centralizing its analysis on behavior, it is possible to elaborate a Sequential Plan of Action (PSA), aiming to act on behavior based on the behaviorist formula ($^{SD}$ - R# - R/Renforcement +/-). The R# is equivalent to the different functions in the response to the discriminatory stimulus).

The method based on ABA as an intervention proposal, mainly in children with signs and symptoms of Autism Spectrum Disorder has in its most significant contribution the elaboration of a curriculum that meets the specific needs of the child's social life and it is in this segment that PSA becomes a descriptive and explanatory tool of how to structure the environment for adaptability to be achieved. In the curriculum to be followed there is a sequence of selection, this sequencing being developed by language, social, personal (basic care), play and motor skills. There is in academic skills a parameter of the ideal to be related. Thus, actions will be planned from basic to complex.

The intensity of the workload to be carried out between 20 and 27 hours per week (complementary with integrative activities) over a minimum period of 24 months extends to the commitment of the parents in the execution of the tasks and the involvement of the family in the elaboration of PSA so that the use of methodologies (TTD, Teaching by Discrete Attempts, CV, Verbal Behaviour, TRD, Teaching by Dynamic Response, and EI, Incidental Teaching) is selected according to the need and specificity of the child. The movement to include other dynamics or even the change in the increase or decrease of intervention intensity is analysed by the monitor/teacher together with the family or caregivers. The success at each stage is in this collaboration.

The concern with the levels of difficulty of each task makes it possible to set up programmes that unfold into tasks. These programmes range from basic oral hygiene care (PCH) to the achievement of an illusionary act of speech. Auditory and visual *feedback* are components of receptive language, which in genesis corresponds to the ability to understand the spoken word. Reciprocity between reception and expression is inseparable, but in neurodevelopmental disorders, where there are significant deficits in language, it is necessary to ensure that the stage prior to the use of the sign is fulfilled, what was planned to be said (level of understanding).

The ability to express oneself in a non-verbal or verbal manner is called expressive language. The expression initially presupposes reception, because after the understanding of concepts and the composition of signs, but not always the two indexes of languages are impaired in a disorder. There may then be a deficit in expressive capacity only, with reception remaining undamaged.

The expression presupposes reception. However, reception can be intact if only the expression is deficient (SOARES, 2005).

In an evaluation of the receptive and expressive capacity of language, it is important to evaluate the intrinsic aspects of each instance of reception or expression, even if there are assumptions between them.

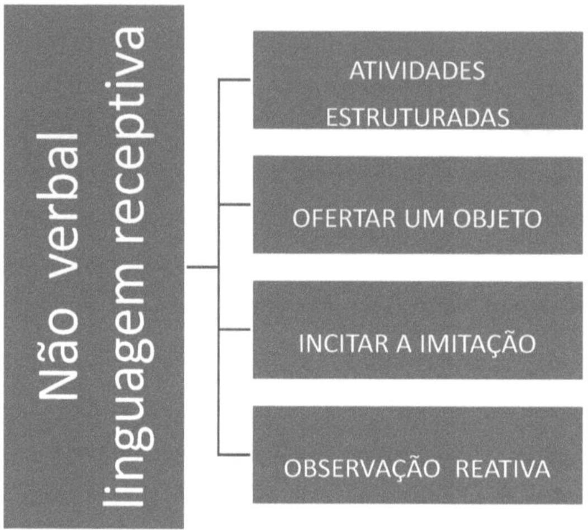


Source: Brazilian Association of Psychosomatic Medicine-MT/2020

# EVALUATION

In assessing the aspects of receptive language, we will start structuring activities by segmented and sequential tasks:

**HB - Skill: Playing**

1. Presentation of a toy for the child and observe its reaction to the offer.
2. Repeat command/imitation of action models.

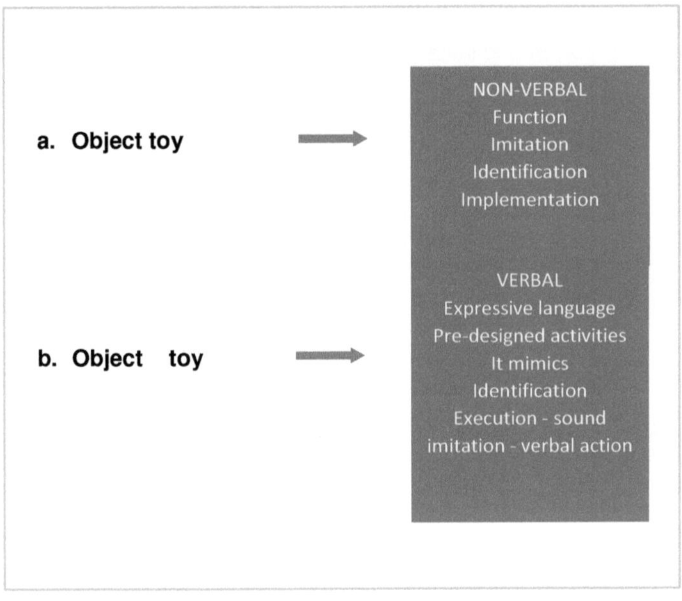



Source: Brazilian Association of Psychosomatic Medicine-MT/2020

## EVALUATION OF COMMUNICATIVE SKILLS: VERBAL AND NON-VERBAL

| Verbal<br>**Non-verbal**<br>Cutting: Ability to make at least 3 hits on a set of evaluated items. | **Expressive language**<br>Pre-designed activities;<br>Observation of sounds and words;<br>Responsiveness;<br>Responsive behaviour. | **Receptive language**<br>Structured activities;<br>Present object;<br>Analyse reaction;<br>Imitation/repeat command. |
|---|---|---|
| **Equivalence** | **Items assessed** | **Items assessed** |
| Scale<br><br>A – 1<br>B – 2<br>C – 3<br>D – 4<br>E – 5<br>F – 6 | Sound imitation<br>Imitation of simple words<br>Name production<br>Verb imitation/verbal action<br>Starting conversation<br>Sentence production with two words | Toy/functional object<br>Engine<br>Imitation<br>Identification of objects<br>Figure identification<br>Performance of tasks |
| **Criteria:**<br>**Communicative Skills** | **Criteria: V.1 - Verbal** | **Criteria: V.2 - Not Verbal** |

Source: Brazilian Association of Psychosomatic Medicine-MT/2020

TTD/TDT or DTT - Discrete Attempts Teaching is one of the ABA method methods of intervening in the signs and symptoms of Autistic Spectrum Disorder. The sequencing of tasks in detailed steps of small blocks of knowledge about the social environment, and at each step by a series of sensitive attempts with initially discreet changes in social, personal, motor, play and language behaviour of the child is the procedural route of this methodology.

An example of Teaching by Discreet Attempts is that it needs to participate in a dynamic that requires social behavioural competence and chair-dancing motor skills and that for academic behaviour of social ability and interaction the motor behaviour of standing, running, stopping and sitting, these four movements should be trained one by one at each specific stage so that the singular movement is acquired and then each one is sequentialised and related.

If the child does not yet issue these behaviours separately, there is no point in a positive reinforcement in sequencing the four behaviours to this desired academic behaviour. (Participating in the chair dance game - Play). It is necessary, then, to emit the behaviour of standing up. And the training to acquire this behaviour goes from the balance application and motor coordination.

The advantage of having one by one in the process of applying this method provides safety and acuity in the development of tasks that may suggest the participation of the monitor/teacher that will help if the child does not have the balance or physically has some damage that produces more difficulty in motor action. In the first attempts, a series of physical interventions of collaboration and physical help may emerge, but as the monitor/teacher or applicator of the programme perceives evolution and gradual decrease of the difficulty in the emission of the behaviour, it should offer a positive (arbitrary) reinforcement for the gradual increase in the frequency of this behaviour. But how to proceed in order to sediment this behaviour? It is in the exhaustive and continuous repetition in which the behaviour will be acquired without the need for physical collaboration of the applicator autonomously.

It is important to always take into account that the focus is on activities structured by positive reinforcement strategies, with reward and motivation. Even when designing the curriculum in PSA, HL - Language Skills, the focus should still be on positive reinforcement. Verbal Behaviour (CV) is a methodology of work that is very similar to the purpose of TTD, for its intensity and sequencing. What is specific is the purpose of the relationship between language and linguistic meaning/concept. This meaning can later be extended to the broad and stricto sense. Later, indices and patterns of functionality and evolution of the echo, tact, command, receptive, RFCC and intraverbal will be presented, which are called verbal operants.

Incidental Teaching is based on interactions between children and adults naturally in routine situations, with the aim of developing new communication skills (Risley and Hart/1975). It is therefore necessary to propose a reorganization of the activities based on natural and facilitating environments, and the adaptation of the environment would provide the favourable conditions for teaching. The interest of the child in the proposal of incidental teaching is the driver of the results planned in PSA. This type of teaching in a natural environment is based on the attribution of meanings and meanings to the real activities of the child in a space that presents itself as a motivating factor for the development of skills. A natural element contributes to the generalization, thus strengthening the simulated transfers in this environment for the child's daily life.

Dynamic Response Teaching is a partially structured methodology, with natural opportunities, one can insert its most motivating factor of intervention. The areas of attention are from child self-initiation, autonomy, protagonism, self-management, and the condition of response to various mobilizations and especially motivation. The *Pivotal Response Training* has, thus, its most effective occurrence in natural environments, with changes of shifts and activities, exercises and tasks already recognized and partially learned.

The study of how an individual interacts and relates with the environment, read in this guideline, any environment, is the object of the study of behaviorist behaviorism. Thus, the interactions between the responses of individuals and the stimulations of the environment make possible in this action a behavioral reading capable of analysis. And it is in this analysis of this behavior resulting from this interaction that we act in the elaboration of a sequential action plan (PSA) in the child in the Autistic Spectrum Disorder.

Acting on the resulting force (behaviour) of the interaction between a child's way of doing something and the environment in which its response (doing) takes place is the proposal of this method. The analysis of the interaction between the child and his environment, between his actions or responses and his environment or stimuli is the intended orientation towards a particular response and a specific stimulus for reinforcement. The set of stimuli (stimulations/environment) and the response (actions/doing) of a child that are related is what we call child behaviour, for the purpose of analysis and action of PSA.

| Behaviour | | |
|---|---|---|
| **Stimulus Discriminatory**<br>SD | **Response**<br>**R#** | **Consequence**<br>**R+/-** |

Source: School of Health in Psychosomatic Medicine - ESMP/2020

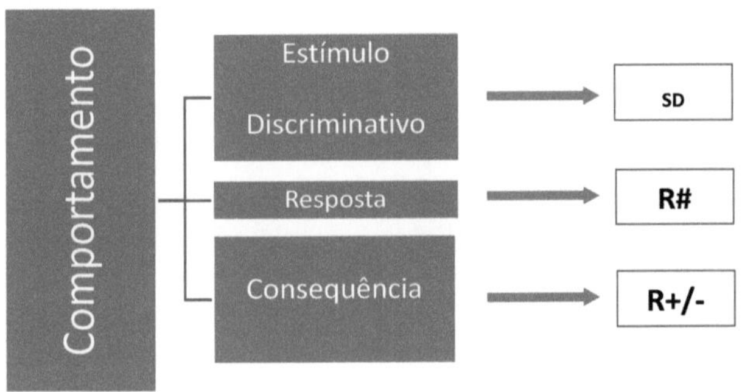


Source: School of Health in Psychosomatic Medicine - ESMP/2020

| PROGRAMME STRATEGIES - TAB | | |
|---|---|---|
| **Item** | **Nomenclature** | **Concept** |
| 1 | Stimulation - **SD** Discriminatory | The beginning of the command to be given or the preceding initial instruction that directs the initial speech or presentation of various contents and material resources is called a discriminatory stimulus. It is of an illogical nature. (It is usually a verbal command preceded by a non-verbal model) |

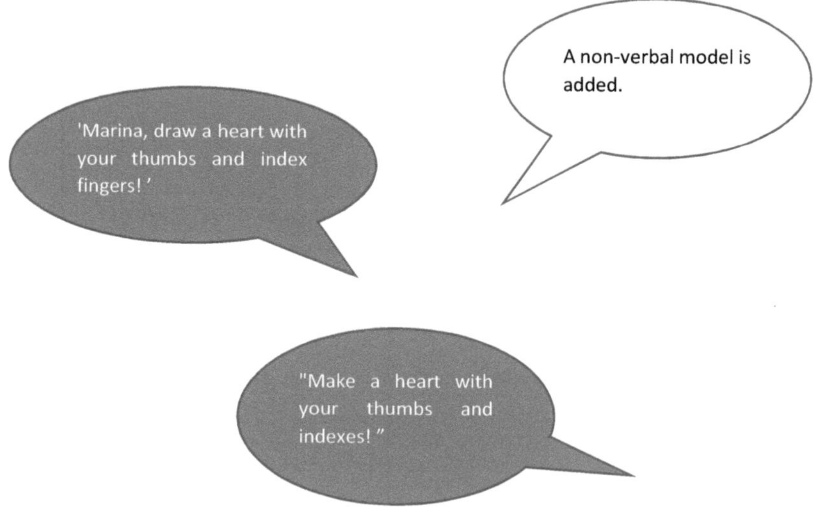

| PROGRAMME STRATEGIES - TAB | | |
| --- | --- | --- |
| **Item** | **Nomenclature** | **Concept** |
| 2 | Attempt - Ta | The presentation of an $SD$ in a complete sequence, achieving a response and the reinforcing consequence of the response. During the session time an operating conditioning unit is required. This basic unit used in the session is Ta. |

**ABA programme for play behaviour skills:**

**HCB1 - play in yellow.**

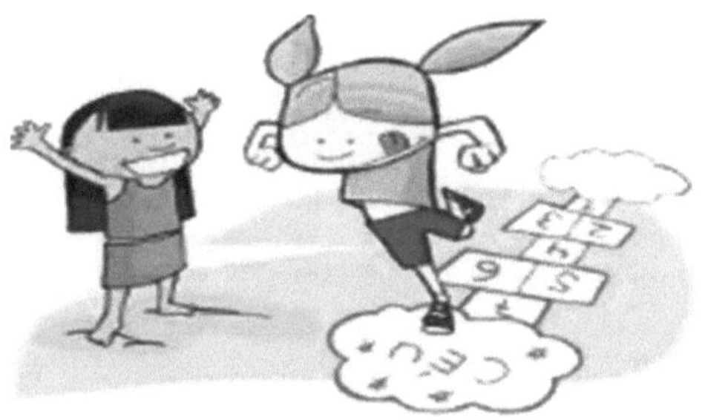

**Applicator:** "Renata, skip the board/field".

Initial verbal command - the request to skip the board/field.

*acressure non-verbal command

**Applicator:** "Renata, you jumped very well, congratulations! The applier claps"

The applicator goes to the child and helps him/her to jump the other fields on his/her side.

"Excellent, Renata!

| PROGRAMME STRATEGIES - TAB | | |
|---|---|---|
| **Item** | **Nomenclature** | **Concept** |
| 3 | Answer - R | To an expected or acceptable behaviour (response) in the proposed relational and dimensional patterns in question. |

**ABA programme for social skills behaviour:**

**HS1 - playing with his little friends.**

**Applicator:** "Daughter, your little friends would be happy if you went and played with them".

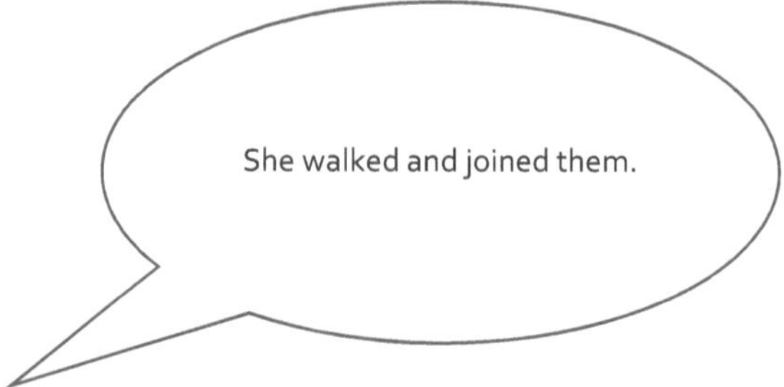

**Applicator:** 'You see, child! (And smiled.)

<table>
<tr><td colspan="3" align="center">PROGRAMME STRATEGIES - TAB</td></tr>
<tr><td>Item</td><td>Nomenclature</td><td>Concept</td></tr>
<tr><td>4</td><td>Booster - $^{SR}$</td><td>The abbreviation "booster stimulus" can be extended to "$^{SR+}$", also referred to as a consequence that follows a response and is thus a booster. The consequence may be positive or not and it is its strength (operant conditioning) that will determine the repetition or not of this behaviour in other situations.</td></tr>
</table>

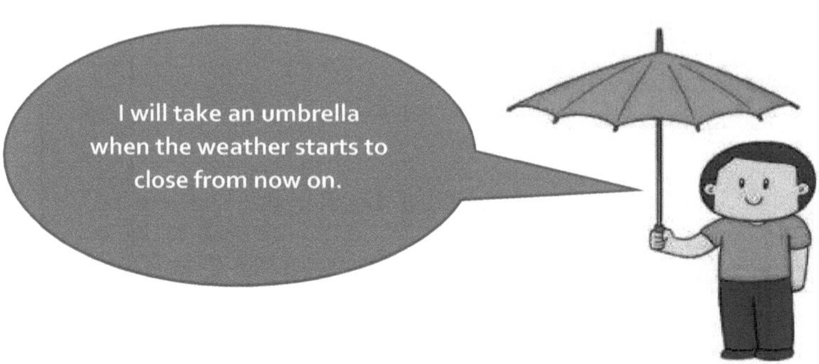



| PROGRAMME STRATEGIES - TAB | | |
|---|---|---|
| Item | Nomenclature | Concept |
| 5 | Contribution/help | The contribution of the monitor or applicator of the programme with additional help or tips or additional information that can be used during the execution of the tasks and the performance. |

<table>
<tr><th colspan="3">PROGRAMME STRATEGIES - TAB</th></tr>
<tr><th>Item</th><th>Nomenclature</th><th>Concept</th></tr>
<tr><td>6</td><td>Stimuli</td><td>The set of inputs that can be used for the development of a program or even task or action that range from concrete materials, figures, cards blocks and other objects that have the nature of acting in a response.</td></tr>
</table>

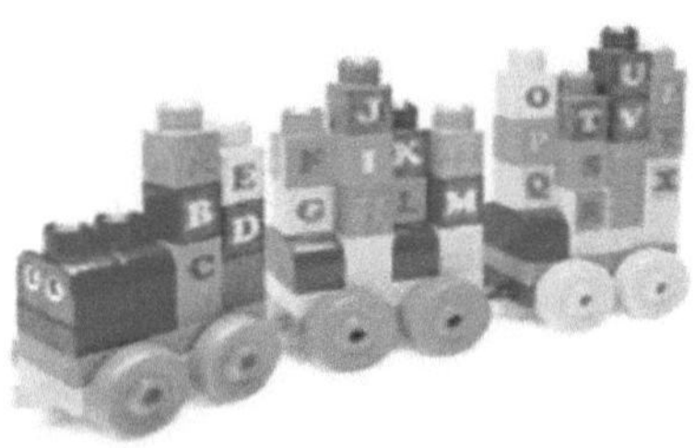

<table>
<tr><th colspan="3">PROGRAMME STRATEGIES - TAB</th></tr>
<tr><th>Item</th><th>Nomenclature</th><th>Concept</th></tr>
<tr><td>7</td><td>Session</td><td>The sequence of time in which therapeutic activities are developed with the child.</td></tr>
</table>

| PROGRAMME STRATEGIES - TAB | | |
|---|---|---|
| **Item** | **Nomenclature** | **Concept** |
| 8 | Domain | The fluency that contemplates the whole learning to be operationalized in the task of the program CV/10 attempts executed in and successive sessions/classes - equivalence of 80%. Basic criteria that make it possible to measure the level of learning of skills and their readiness for the consequent levels and tasks. |

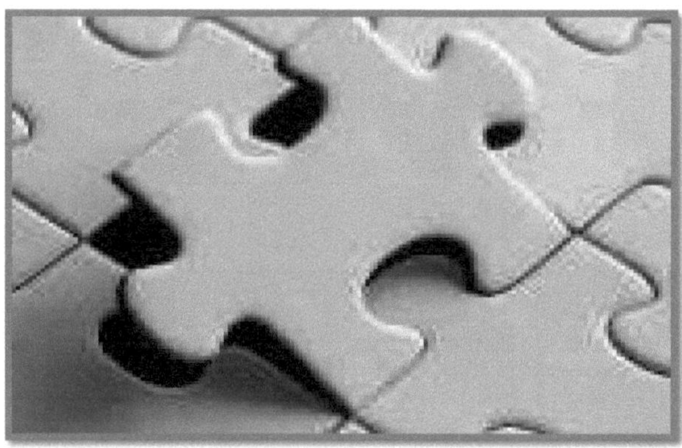

| PROGRAMME STRATEGIES - TAB | | |
|---|---|---|
| **Item** | **Nomenclature** | **Concept** |
| 9 | Data | The set of information and records of a child's actions in attempts, hits and errors or even gaps (lack of answers) or approach to the objective of the task. The responses to the discriminatory stimulus vary from correct ('+' / '√') / incorrect ('-'or an 'x') / no response (NR / SR) / approach ('A' or 'S' for successive approach). |

| PROGRAMME STRATEGIES - TAB | | |
|---|---|---|
| **Item** | **Nomenclature** | **Concept** |
| 10 | Method and methodologies | The sequential and detailed description of the specific material/task/action presentation phases, with their respective structured spaces and functional structure. |

| NET Education in Natural Environments | | |
|---|---|---|
| **FCC** Functions, Features and Classes | | |
| **REINFORCING ACTIVITY** | **APPLICATOR'S STIMULUS** | **SKILLS** Receptive, tactful, verbal, intraverbal command. |
| MUSIC | What is this music? | Tact |
| CELLULAR | What colour is this phone? / What does it do? | Intraverbal |
| ANA HOLIDAYS | Point to the CD. What is this? | Tact |
| ANA HOLIDAYS | Say: Let's go to the pool. | Ecoico |
| TURN | What can we do for fun in the pool? | Intraverbal |
| PRACTICAL ACTIVITIES | Show me how you jump? | Receptive |
| PRACTICAL ACTIVITIES | What is the tyre doing? (Rotating) | Intraverbal |
| PRACTICAL ACTIVITIES | What have I done with the bike? (I crashed) | Intraverbal |

**Source: ABMP/Centre West/2020**

NET / Natural Environment Education is carried out in spaces that allow the development of activities in the natural environment. It does not have a table or a sequence of objects, equipment or adapted space. This does not mean that there is no planning. The idea is to select a natural and spontaneous reinforcement environment in order to develop the skills in the classes / play sessions. The orientation is that the activities are as less structured as possible, with interventions being introduced in natural and reinforcing situations. There are two very important strategies in this orientation. The first is called Advance Planning, **i.e. to** be sure of what the child really likes. A space that he feels comfortable, a park, a football field, a walking track, or even a square. The most effective reinforcement is his presence. Always make use of it.

| ABA PROGRAMME | | |
|---|---|---|
| **CURRICULUM** | | |
| **ACTIVITY** | **APPLICATOR'S STIMULUS** | **STIMULES** |
| Receptive language 1 | Touching different body parts | Head, shoulders, knees, toes. |
| Receptive language 2 | Playing a common item | Book, crayon, SpongeBob, Lego piece. |
| Visual performance | Pair equal figures | 10 pairs of figures |
| Imitation | Imitating movements with objects | Various |
| Vocal imitation | Imitate words when requested | Cake, juice, bear, car, yes, no. |
| Appointment | Naming common objects | DVD, book, cup, blanket, car. |
| Intraverbal | Complete song words | "Palm, palm, palm" "Ciranda, cirandinha". |

**(LEAR, K.2004)**

Robert Koegel presented in his work a method that would later work as an intervention, through teaching and learning skills in natural situations: the *Pivoltal Response Treatment* or Dynamic Response Training. This intervention is naturalistic because it relates to the dynamic environment without a very fixed structure. Activities are learned based on opportunities and consequences, observing the gradual and exponential increase of motivation, with tasks, interleaving and choices.

## LANGUAGE SKILLS: RECEPTIVE AND EXPRESSIVE LANGUAGE

Changes in language acquisition, whether due to a similar chronology or to late development in learning, are the most frequent complaints regarding signs, symptoms, disorders and neurodevelopment disorders. This clinical reality is a worrying factor for the various segments that articulate themselves in the neuro-typical referential of childhood development.

Language is the prognosis of Autistic Spectrum Disorder. Thus, the development of language is based on two fundamental axes of superior cortical function: anatomofunctional structure and verbal stimulation. The distinction lies in the determining nature of biology and the influence of external environment and conditions. It is important for the knowledge and recognition of the neurobiological bases of language to consider it as being processed in different anatomical structures.

The bioelectric studies of brain tissue and the most different imaging techniques allow a more comprehensive study of the neurophysiology of language, because both speech, understanding, reception and nomination can suffer natural or biologically determined damage.

The basic principle has left hemisphere predominance for language development, according to Kandel (2003), language processing in about 96% of people is carried out in this hemisphere. An important issue corroborating the clinical study in question proposed by Broca in 1864 is Wada's test, which qualitatively and quantitatively assesses laterality and verbal functions, both with respect to language and its memory.

In this clinical examination, the application of an anaesthetic to the left cerebral hemisphere usually blocks speech. The associative areas of the cerebral cortex, two cortical areas which do not normally perform their functions, correspond to significant losses in language, a *sine qua non* condition to exclude the motor and sensory primary or secondary areas of location which control language functions.

For a more descriptive understanding, from the nosographic point of view of the disorders, the areas that will be studied will be called the parieto-occipitotemporal associative area and the pre-frontal associative area. The knowledge of these areas enables a more precise intervention in mapping and complementary practices that could relate to the specificities of these function control plans.

The drill area is in the prefrontal associative area, it is related to the motor cortex for sequentiality planning of movements and it is connected by subcortical fiber bundle to the parieto-occipitotemporal associative area. It has in the area of Broca what we can consider as an indispensable circuit for the formation of the word and is found in the region of the prefrontal cortex.

It can then be said that in the posterolateral prefrontal cortex and in the pre-motor part the motor patterns are planned so that the individual words are expressed naturally and received effectively. The parieto-occipitotemporal associative area is an area for language understanding, object naming, primary lecto-language processing and spatial coordinates of the body with regard to analysis.

The understanding of language and naming of objects is fundamental for the linguistic activities of reception, comprehension and speech to be carried out in the normal way. In the temporal lobe, Wernicke's area is located, with a functional aim of evoking concepts by means of sound processing, which when received and recognised are interpreted as words.

It is in the act of understanding words that the function of Wernicke's area and any injury in this area is based. But the relative association between the Wernicke centre and the Broca area must be considered. The area for naming objects is on the side of the anterior region of the occipital lobe and the posterior region of the temporal lobe.

Vision and hearing are involved in this process, one concerning the learning of names and the other about the physical nature of the object. This realisation is a condition without which language cannot be understood. It is important to consider that even with the polarization of the areas of Wernicke and Broca, reading is a consequence of the integration of the two areas, and this dependence would signal the reception of information from the left visual cortex.

Clinical studies have deepened the mechanism of action, reception, production and understanding of language, and biological cartesianism is not admissible when brain damage or even genetic damage are analysed. New cortical and subcortical regions in the left hemisphere have been involved in this process and are essential for language acquisition and development.

Language implementation systems (Wernicke and Broca, involving insular cortex and base nuclei, with function of afferent auditory signals analysis, phonic construction and articulatory control). This conceptual system, which has the function of basing the conceptual knowledge, being regions distributed among the associative cortex of superior order. And, finally, the mediating system that acts in an intermediary way and constitutes several regions in the frontal, parietal, and temporal association cortex.

Neurons that relate to each other forming a network and are distributed in various regions of the brain are responsible in a specialized way for language processing. It is the hearing aid that is responsible for synchronising the auditory signals and, by decoding them, turning them into electrical impulses. These impulses travel through the neurons to the auditory area of the cerebral cortex in the temporal lobe.

The recognition of auditory signal patterns, interpretation, formulation of concepts or thoughts, with activation of various groups of nerve cells is a specific function of the Wernicke area. In the lower part of the temporal lobe, the image of what acoustic signal is formed, and the related concepts are stored in the parietal lobe. We consider the opposite process for thought verbalization. An internal verbalization is channeled to the Broca area, in the lower part of the frontal lobe, to be effective in speech production. Both the motor control areas and those responsible for memory are involved in language.

It is important to stress that more than 90% of the population is dominated by the left hemisphere for language processing, but the right hemisphere also participates in this processing. Brain damage results in language (speech) and comprehension disorders that are called aphasia, thus impairing the ability to speak and understand speech. Prosody, resonance, articulation, voice, cadence/pace characterise speech.

When the language changes, we can classify them as: deviation, delay and decoupling.

| Language Changes | | | |
|---|---|---|---|
| **Item** | **Diversions** | **Delay** | **Dissociation** |
| 1 | StandardEvolution | ProgressionLanguage | Significant Distinction |
| 2 | Amended | Slower pace | Relationship Areas |
| 3 | AnomalyAcquisitionLanguage | SequenceCorrect | DifferenceEvolution |

**Source: Brazilian Association of Psychosomatic Medicine-MT/2019**

The factors contributing to the etiology of learning and language difficulties and disorders are diverse, whether they are emotional, intellectual or cognitive and organic. There are close relationships between certain disorders and language. It will be specifically treated for Autistic Spectrum Disorder - TEA, however, we can highlight dyslexia, dyslalia, dyscalculia, epilepsy and other aphasia.

The decrease in written or oral language ability resulting from any brain disorder is called aphasia. Disorders of this nature are diverse and there are a multitude of tests, evaluations and reports to classify the types and identify forms of intervention, with priority being given to this in the first years of a child's life.

In general, aphasias are systematized and called sensory and motor, the latter still receives the denomination expressive, because it is closely connected to the difficulty in the production of speech, damaging in terms of rhythm, cadence and fluency. Receptive aphasia, or also called sensory aphasia, most of the time refers to impairments and difficulties in understanding speech and language, impairing reading and writing in aphasic patients.

As a constitutive part of aphasia syndrome, we have speech apraxia. In these patients, more than understanding, reading and writing, motor impairments are perceived, such as specialized disability in orofacial movements. Since the linguistic nature is what definitely marks aphasia, the inability to develop motor is the disorder that produces inefficiency in the prosodic condition, with gaps, spaces and slow fluency, causing misunderstandings in the articulation.

Muscle changes, such as prosody, phonation joint, and resonance, which also involve breathing, are characteristic of the speech disorder called dysarthria. These symptoms have a casuistry in the CNS or Peripheral lesions, with fixation or paralysis in the speech muscles, that is, lack of coordination in muscle control. Even though apraxia and dysarthria are motor disorders of speech, the losses are different at the production level. Fixity/paralysis, lentification, muscle tone are not significant elements in apraxic patients. Ataxia, hypertension or hypotension, restrictive speech muscle movement are specific to dysarthria.

The assessment of the patient's language at various levels of complexity of speech activities, repetition, description, understanding and other constitutive elements of communication and language, in addition to the assessment of the elements that constitute and compete for speech and the movements and tasks involving motor programming.

Studies involving electroencephalographic discharges, seizures, in general, all the symptoms arising from epileptic seizures bring some specific disorders into the current clinical picture of language disorders.

Acute or critical aphasia with transient cognitive dysfunction, Landau-Kleffner Syndrome, or acquired epileptic aphasia, and developmental dysphasia that is clinically related to epilepsy. It is known from clinical grounds that the cause of this aphasia is continuous seizures or activities involving abnormal epileptiform electroencephalography, even if there is often apparent confusion with symptoms of the autistic disorder.

In the case of dyslexia, it is important to note that, according to Rutkowski (2003), there is a significant clinical discrepancy when comparing the data of Brazilian children with those of developed countries, with about 40% of them having difficulties in writing in the early years, and this percentage decreases by half in more developed countries.

The sensory-perceived, socio-emotional, and motor memory are integralities that articulate to the combination of environmental and biological phenomena in terms of quantity, quality, and frequency of stimuli that the environment offers in learning language/communication.

The literature is the basis for the analysis of dyslexia, as it is a significant change in children's learning, differentiating itself from acquisition and development. Acquired dyslexia is the result of brain damage in the biological/ genetic case.

The causes involving the environment or the school space would characterise developmental dyslexia.

Neurological, neuroanatomical and neurophysiological factors, cognition factors, genetic basis, premature birth and others as below average weight would characterize developmental dyslexia. Another division of dyslexia refers to the so-called central and peripheral types. In central dyslexia, there is impairment in the conversion from correct spelling to speech.

In peripheral dyslexia, the commitment is in the understanding of the reading content, that is, more in visual perception. The phonological, surface and deep types are part as subtypes of central dyslexia, while attentional, pure (literal) or negligent are the peripheral dyslexia. Surface, semantic and phonological dyslexia are more common in so-called developmental dyslexia.

Among the central and peripheral dyslexia, we have as clinical foundation of pure or literal dyslexia the letter by letter reading preserved and in the neuroanatomic characteristics occipital lesions inferior to the left. The lesions in the left parietal lobe constitute the neuroanatomic characteristics of attentional dyslexia, and there is preservation of the reading of isolated words, but when grouped, difficulties in reading in the global visual field persist.

The lesion in the middle cerebral artery region of the right hemisphere involving frontal, parietal, frontal and temporal lobes is part of the neuroanatomical characters of neglect dyslexia and the damage to the visual field of the contralateral side of the brain is one of the clinical foundations of this learning change. The clinical characteristics of deep dyslexia are reading fluency for frequent and concrete words, absence of non-word readings, and blockage in the nonlexical pathway.

Multiple lesions in the left hemisphere and the existence of residual reading skills in the right hemisphere are neuroanatomical features of this type of dyslexia. Evidence of dysfunction in the left hemisphere middle and upper-posterior temporal region are neuroanatomical features of surface dyslexia, with clinical features of lexical pathway impairment, without orthographic capacity for information.

The last type is phonological dyslexia, which has a clinical basis of incapacity of phonological decoding, damage to the phoneme-grapheme conversion pathway, difficulties in phonological memory tasks, insufficient performance in reading pseudo-words. Regarding the proper functioning of perilexical processing, no specific neuroanatomical dysfunctions are perceived. Studies that relate dyslexia to genetics consider reading linked to specific chromosomes 6, 1, 2 and 15.

The Human Genome Project lists the DYX1, DYX2, DYX3 and DYX4 dyslexia susceptibility genes. The same specific chromosomes mentioned above have been identified as related to damage in text processing. Changes in written language, be it disortography or dysgraphics, refer respectively to orthographic changes in the spelling of words, with dysgraphics being changes in the strokes of letters. The etiology of oral and written language disorders refer to alterations in hearing, cognitive, autistic, environmental or environmental influence deficits, constitutional or isolated delay in expressive language and other specific alterations in language.

The descriptive analysis of these disorders is based, respectively:

It influences the acquisition of language after 6-9 months, observing the changes in vocal quality loss, suppressed consonants and modification of the sound of vowels. Guttural and primitive sounds still persist.

2. The developmental delay in the development of language in the child is partly similar to that of the normal child, at a rate of involution.

3. Occurrence of ecology, inappropriate persistence of the same theme (perseverance), changes in nonverbal communication, stereotypical and repetitive behaviour, restrictive interests and prejudice to sociability.

4. Elements involving social and emotional risks.

5. Prejudice and delay related to pragmatism and understanding. In the case of other specific language changes, it is a differential diagnosis of exclusion.

# THE MANAGEMENT OF STEREOTYPES

The management of stereotypes is the monitoring and guidance for an intervention that makes it possible to replace one motor behaviour with another that is desired. The term stereotype comes from the Greek *steros,* which means solid, *typos,* model.

Stereotyping is in essence a compulsive defence" (Cantavella et al., 1992).

This work is accurate and demands not only dexterity due to the sensitive nature of the situation involving the child with Autism Spectrum Disorder - TEA/Autism and its specific forms of self-regulation, but also through these movements and the way these children act to regulate themselves and discharge tension. There is no apparent function in these stereotyped and repetitive movements.

It can be said, then, that the so-called repetition, insistence and perseverance in movements should not be extinguished but replaced for an action that also has the same regulatory result as the previous one, but without social harm, that is, more acceptable and that does not incur any kind of physical impact harmful to the child (self-mutilation). Using hands or feet with activities that are compatible with persevering stimuli is a good methodology. The planning of activities by PSA - Curriculum has a good contingency to reduce stereotyped, persevering and repetitive movements when the child has constant motor activities to reduce anxiety. Manual and lower limb activities and fine practice reduce stereotypes through the development of motor exercises.

The cause of these movements is then related to stress, anxiety and irritability. The understanding of relationships and the etiology of these movements: what caused and triggered the stress situation by mobilizing the movements to discharge tension is the mapping capable of identifying other ways of expressing excitement. The reduction of attention, whether voluntary in which the voluntary desire to fix on something is present, or spontaneous, with other stimuli standing out over attention, making the child hypotenous, with the gradual decrease of attention, called hypoprosexia or aprosexia, is a harmful factor in the operationalization of knowledge in the occurrence of stereotypes. According to Sanger (2010), the duration of stereotyping is variable and can occur for seconds, minutes, and even hours if the child is not distracted by another activity.

The understanding of relationships and socio-emotional reciprocity aggregated to communicative behaviour are clinical criteria for psychopathological diagnosis in Autism Spectrum Disorder - TEA/Autism. Knowing the adherence and fixity, which present themselves as insistence on sameness, inflexible adherence to routines, ritualized patterns of verbal behavior, rigid patterns of thought and fixed and restricted interests, abnormality and intensity and focus attachment to uncommon, circumscribed and persevering interests can have their impacts minimized from a sequential plan of action of apparent predictability in the routine, the use of rules previously presented and understood and space with structured environment, with methodologies of constant and meaningful activities.

Impeded to appeal to language and without imaginary articulation that allows them to perceive things in the world in the same way as their fellow men, they produce symptoms with their bodies (gestural stereotypes, "rocking", "flapyng", and other ritual and repetitive movements) in the attempt to, through repetition, structure a minimum of organization for their lives. (SIBEMBERG, 1998, p. 65).

| Management of Stereotypes | | | |
|---|---|---|---|
| **Item** | **Stereotypes** | **Symptoms** | **Intervention** |
| 1 | Ecolalia | Repetition | Roadmap/model technique |
| 2 | Flapping | Movement of senior members | Replacement by desirable and socially acceptable activities |
| 3 | Rocking | Balance/gauge itself/fixing on circular/rotating objects | Micromanagement and substitutive behaviours (sports) |

**Source: Brazilian Association of Psychosomatic Medicine-MT/2020.**

Regulatory actions are also neuro-typical behaviors. In other words, physiologically they can be part of the acquisition of language and, also, in the motor acquisition in rhythm and gait, however they lose their strength in the first months of life and tend to disappear until the age of 3 (three), leaving a few behaviors in search of physical sensation (sensory regulation), in school years. According to Fernandez-Alvarez (2003), self-stimulatory behaviours tend to decrease from six months of age and according to Thelen (1979), they disappear at the age of 3. So, it can be said that turning objects, curling hair or even continuously swinging legs are behaviours that we usually perform in our daily life, with the aim of alleviating our anxiety, reducing stress and the discharge of a feeling of relief. As well as snapping our fingers reduces the accumulation of tension, stereotyped movements or motor behaviours with a repetitive character (DSM 5) are part of the self-regulation and search for physical sensation in Autism Spectrum Disorder.

Stereotypes are, therefore, motor behaviours with a repetitive, apparently impulsive character and without motive (Criterion A), and are generally rhythmic of the head, hands or body without an apparent adaptive function (DSM 5/2013). The function of these movements is related to the organisation, reassurance (calmness) and reorganisation and multimodality of boosters. According to Laver (2001), multimodality is the occurrence within scenes of joint attention, and involves components beyond speech, such as looking and gestures.

Contrary to popular belief, then, this behaviour is more common than it appeared to be. The search for sensory regulation, relief from everyday anxiety and the reduction of stress, not to mention irritability, which can arise from a day-to-day environmental stimulus, rush-hour traffic. What would be the difference for the child in TEA/Autism and the typical?

The answer would be in the field: frequency, duration and intensity of these behaviours, as well as the level of commitment in the social, family, school and professional fields. The fact that the child performs these movements without an apparently specific purpose (he moves because he feels the physical need to perform the movement) makes the focus not on exclusion from the stereotype but on its replacement for a more desirable and socially accepted behaviour.

From this decontextualisation, one can deduce the damage to the child's attention (hypoprosexia or hypotenacity), at the moment when the child's natural environment and the dislocation of the child to motor behaviour take place. The distraction is thus the result of the demand for self-regulation and sensory search, which also makes it possible to analyse that their best form of intervention is in this incursion of physical sensation. The Analysis of Applied Behavior - ABA has in its academic skills to be developed (personal/care, play, language, motor and social) an important set of actions carried out in the sequential action plan, with a well adapted curriculum, which enables the intervention, with a substitute and Micromanagement view, in these situations, with modeling, sensory integration, imitation, scripts and language stimulation.

The environment can also be conceived in a multimodal way, in a set of verbal and non-verbal activities that exceed the child's capacity for reception, causing an overload of sensations and feelings in this excessive apprehension. The discharge of tension results in these movements, being an escape from this accumulation of sensations, in the search for sensory regulation. The hypersensitivity of some children (restriction to colour, shapes, textures, food, avoidance diet, sounds and tissues). In the case of sensory search, it is the behaviour that insists on various sensory experiences (sniffing, spinning, biting, fixation on lights, circular and spinning objects). It is important to point out that by attaching oneself to these actions and objects which enable a discharge of self-pleasure and self-regulation, the child integrates this pattern as a repertoire of fixation, insistence and perseverance. What is most effective in ABA is the undoing of this repertory of fixation, integrating and reintegrating behaviors that are desirable, strengthening socio-emotional reciprocity and the understanding of relationships. The Sequential Plan of Action, with its adapted and semi-structured or structured curriculum, has as its functionality the viability of social interaction activities, the opportunity of new experiences and diversified spaces to increase the repertoire of specific knowledge for its subsequent generalization and the substitution of stereotyped behaviors that are undesirable and harmful to children. It is important to stress that intervention activities should be sequenced and detailed. Any work that is of extreme and violent disruption has the opposite effect, making it possible to increase the FDI of the domain - Frequency, Duration and Intensity.

Ritualized actions are also called repetitive and are the result of excessive motor movements, communicative behaviour and postural consciousness. The self-regulatory movements in TEA/Autism have a function of reorganization and processing and operationalization of physical sensations. This sensory regulation is in addition to a discharge of self-pleasure, relieving the excess of stimuli and reducing stress and anxiety, so it contributes in the moment it calms down and reorganizes.

| Item | Repetitive or ritualistic actions |
|---|---|
| 1 | Rotate around you - Turn objects or rotate around your axis |
| 2 | Fixation on objects that turn or are luminous |
| 3 | Balance of upper limbs - hands and arms and forearms |
| 4 | Movement of hands in front of face or eyes |
| 5 | Continuous repetition of sounds or part of words |
| 6 | Body Balance Forward and Backward |
| 7 | Moving from one side to the other without contingency |
| 8 | Restlessness in lower limbs - feet and legs (cross) |
| 9 | Walking on tiptoe or with your heel off the surface |
| 10 | Jump, run and jump frequently, intensity and duration in an apparent manner |
| 11 | Snapping fingers or even snapping other parts of the body joint |

**Source: Brazilian Association of Psychosomatic Medicine-MT/2020.**

Stereotyping can be a discharge of self-pleasure, self-regulation and the search for physical sensations, however, it is important to point out that a significant frequency of self-stimulation causes aprosexia and global hypotenacity, because the attention is weakened because the child is focused on repetitive or ritualized actions, responding significantly to internal stimuli, and social contact is impaired by stereotypes, reducing the potentiality of social relationships and interaction with the surrounding environment. What to do then? The most effective intervention is in the PSA/Curriculum that potentializes the academic skills the bridge to prevent and reduce repetitive acts, thus replacing the stimuli with desired and socially accepted behaviors, i.e., that meets the practical social functions and aspects of sensory regulation: "calm down, regulate and reorganize".

| Management of Stereotypes | | | |
|---|---|---|---|
| **Restricted and repetitive standards** | | | |
| **Item** | **Background** | **Symptoms** | **Narrative** |
| 1 | Non Verbal | Rocking | Turning in itself (own axis) |
| 2 | Visual | Fixed interests | Visual fascination by moving lights and rotating objects. |
| 3 | Non Verbal | Flapping | Movement of upper limbs and motor repetitive acts with the hands. |

**Source: Brazilian Association of Psychosomatic Medicine-MT/2020.**

The PSA/Curriculum has in the functional evaluation an excellent planning methodology for the determination of a behaviour. The methods of conducting functional evaluation (indirect evaluation, direct observation and experimental manipulations) provide a significant systematization of the monitoring of the management of stereotypes with periodic information, anticipated occurrence of the problem behavior, description of the behavior and occurrence after the behavior. In the "Behaviour" space, the target and problem behaviours will be described, and in the "Background" should contain the hypothetical background, with knowledge gaps (spaces for additions of findings). The teaching consists of both teaching and learning, as critical, social and complex practice between teacher and learner. In the case of the management of stereotypes, the substitutive behaviors should correspond to the physical sensory search and the social function of the proposed activity in the curriculum, by means of elaborated itineraries and micromanagement of the introduction of daily activities that can meet the social needs of children. In this case, positive reinforcement is important, but must be varied.

| Management of Stereotypes | | | |
|---|---|---|---|
| Motor movements: Use of objects in an inappropriate way; stereotyped or repetitive speech, echolalia and idiosyncratic phrases; simple motor stereotyping, aligning toys or rotating objects - Diagnostic Criteria B1 - DSM 5(2013). | | | |
| **Causes** | | | |
| Item | Background | Nature | Intervention/replacement behaviour |
| 1 | Altered sensory stimulation - Diagnostic Criteria B4 - DSM 5 (2013). | Hyper or hyperreactivity - Deficit of a physiological nature that makes it impossible to receive, decode, receive and express sensory stimuli. Sensory stimuli of unusual interest for sensory aspects; apparent indifference to pain/temperature; reaction contrary to sounds or textures and visual fascination with light or movement. | Roadmap, Micromanagement (desensitization) and substitute behaviors. |
| 2 | Restriction in the children's repertoire (socio-emotional reciprocity; communicative behaviour and understanding of relationships.). Diagnostic criteria A1 and A2 and A3 - DSM 5 (2013) | Abnormal social approach, impaired social responses, reduced sharing of interests and affections, impaired verbal communication, variation of the verbal and nonverbal communication deficit poorly integrated with the abnormality. | Replacement by desirable and socially accepted activities - diverse and interdisciplinary games between verbal, non-verbal and paraverbal (self-knowledge). |

| 3 | Ritualised patterns of repetitive behaviour (insistence on sameness and fixed interests - Diagnostic Criteria B2 and B3 - DSM 5 (2013). | Unyielding adherence to routines; ritualized patterns of verbal behaviour; rigid patterns of thinking and eating the same food daily; restricted interests, abnormality and intensity and focus; attachment to unusual objects, circumscribed and persevering interests. | Micromanagement and substitutive behaviors (sports) - games. |
|---|---|---|---|

**Source: Brazilian Association of Psychosomatic Medicine-MT/2020.**

| Management of Stereotypes |
|---|
| **Restrictive and repetitive standards** |
| Rocking motor behaviour - rotating objects or unusual interests for things in rotating movements - Motor motions - Diagnostic Criteria B[1] - DSM 5 (2013). |
| Visual intervention - Use of cards or images with the spinning top. Children playing ciranda. Image of a scooter and exchange of clues and visual codes for image decoding. |
| Intervention: ABA/academic ability Play, ABA/academic ability and ABA/academic motor skills. |
| Present as HB the spinning top and interact with the child so that there is a social function related to the activity. By playing the second game of ciranda-cirandinha develop the motor coordination of fine praxia (holding hands) and balance, giving the game a function of socialization and socio-emotional reciprocity, as well as humming the song, develops the HL, by visual contact and by the repetition/imitation. To present the bambolê, which would be as much for *rocking* as for *flapping* with the hands (forearm), being specific of the *flapping* game of lego or puzzle for neurological effectiveness. |
| Domain: FDI - The domain is of fluent character, in view of being of inconstant frequency. It can appear frequently or in situations of stress or excitement. The outstanding stimuli are responsible for the need to manage anxiety, stress, irritability, excitement and other sensory stimulation needs. |

| Item | Background | Symptoms | Narrative |
|---|---|---|---|

| | | | |
|---|---|---|---|
| 1 | Non Verbal | Rocking | Turning in itself (own axle) / Coarse motor activity. |
| 2 | Visual | Fixed interests | Visual fascination by lights and rotating objects in motion/subtle activities. |
| 3 | Non Verbal | Flapping | Movement of upper limbs and motor repetitive acts with the hands / manipulation of objects. |

**Source: Brazilian Association of Psychosomatic Medicine-MT/2020.**

# PSYCHOSOMATICS AND PSYCHOMOTRICITY

The understanding of the relational binomial health and disease in psychosomatics is quite distinct from psychopathology of an operational-pragmatic nature. The concept of the biopsychosocial subject is very relevant when dealing with the subject who has the illness and not the illness that affects the subject.

Thus, studies in psychosomatics are based on their basic premises and their practical use, which goes back to the principles of Hippocrates. But how do we define psychosomatics? The nuclear concept is relational because it is a system made up of three subsystems: mind, body, and social relationships.

The novelty of this study is in the practical-utilitarian and transdisciplinary sense of the relationship between mind, body and social relationships. It is important to point out that the core of its guidelines is medical-clinical indoctrination, although its transdisciplinary nature has been widely presented, mainly in the seasonality of the social transformations of this pandemic movement (2020) and in the mobilization of the dialectics of meaning of the human sciences.

I begin the discussion about psychosomatics through the brain pole, which is, according to our north of psychosomatic study, the smallest constitutive part of this novel, but it is necessary to understand the foundation of the neurosciences to relate to this constitutive interweaving of human and, indissociably, relational equilibrations and meanings. I would say, then, that there is a trail that leads to the tissue that will be established and formed, according to its constitution imbricated in human subjectivity.

In the brain orientation, then, we have the neurons, which are brain/nerve cells constituent of the brain. It is these cells that through the neurotransmitters communicate, enabling our actions and attitudes. It is important to clarify that psychosomatics is a system that presents three subsystems: mind, which is internal and of introjection and interiorization, body (motricity/psychomotricity) and social relationships, that is, it is in this inter-relationship that we base our line of thought and elaborate our considerations.

Neurotransmitters are substances produced by neurons. When there is excitation of the axon of the presynaptic neuron the neurons are released. When released the neurons move through the synapse to the cell that will be excited or inhibited. When there is a loss, excess or any dysfunction, this imbalance of production is the main reference for disorders such as depression. We cite depression as part of a psychic structure (neurosis) and not as a disorder for psychopathological and diagnostic elaboration of a specific case.

Thus, in the constitution of the brain, we have the neurons, which if they do not react as they should, would result in depression. There are various possibilities of undesirable reactions ranging from stressful experiences and traumatic experiences to alcohol and drug abuse, genetic predisposition, melancholy and diseases in the brain, which are difficult to detect.

The context suggests the disease as a traumatic and degrading situation, but it is from the moment the organism has access to the information that physical wear begins. An example of this is what we call stress, having the possibility to be originated in depression, resulting in several symptoms among them, ulcer and gastritis.

Anhedonia, which is the loss of the capacity to feel pleasure, together with avolution and affective bluntness are characteristic of depression, lack of will to do everyday things, lack of appetite, insomnia and discouragement, as well as hypersonia and increased appetite are symptoms that appear when the depressive process is triggered.

Another symptom of this process is the elaboration of negative thoughts and the symptoms of obsession and compulsion. This combination of symptoms evolved from various disorders has a systemic effect, which because it is diffuse becomes difficult to control and follow its etiology, making its cause-effect relationship hidden and difficult.

We will continue our orientation from the depression, which follows this kind of symptomatic path. Stress gives way to or even articulates with anxiety, resulting in panic attacks, palpitations, refluxes, sweating and headaches without an apparent clinical basis. It is important to emphasize that the fact that no clinical explanation is found does not rule out the evolution of signs and symptoms, thus making the identification of an origin or etiology even more diffuse.

This absence of a specific point, with this characterization in several parts of the organism gives space to the intestinal cycle of constipation (intestinal constipation) and frequent bowel movements. There is also a dermal change and weakening of hair and nails in this cycle. The presence of elements that in a concatenated way trigger other symptoms and wear denotes clinical complexity.

As much as there are tendencies that support one particular form or another of treatment, with a view to psychosomatics being based on an analysis of a single system related to three subsystems: body, mind and social relationships, orientation is a combined form of treatment and interventions, which have as their direction the subject and not the illness or disorder that affects the subject.

The causes are treated by sessions, analysis or therapies, which can be psychoanalytical marked by the seven schools of thought (Freud, Lacan, Bion, Klein, Winnicott, Hartman, Kohut) and the object of psychoanalysis (unconscious) or devices (Oedipus Complex, Narcissism and Mirror Stadium), with a view to the traumatic contents experienced in childhood and reminiscences (sensitive experience transposed to the world of ideas).

## MECHANISM OF SYMPTOM FORMATION: THE BRAIN

In most traumatic situations, the patient's context is responsible for the beginning of the stressful process, however these exophoric/external (degrading) causes give rise to a lack of balance in brain biochemical activity.

From this beginning, the organism takes on the wear and tear and the disease can extend to other important organs and the process of illness evolves. The pituitary gland in conjunction with the hypothalamus and amygdala receives the hazard information and enhances the warning. The information exchanged between them results in the forwarding of impulses and chemical flags.

The alert is reached by the adrenal glands which, as a reaction, releases the neurotransmitter adrenaline or epinephrine, which is a sympathomimetic hormone and has the function of preparing the body for effort and great activities that demand excessive expenditure of energy, with marked acceleration of the heartbeat.

After the increase of the heartbeat, it is the moment of the effort of the lungs to oxygenate the body and follow the rhythm of the heart acceleration. This extra work causes nerve cells to be clamped for the release of noradrenaline.

Noradrenaline or norepinephrine is also a hormone synthesized by the adrenal gland. When released, this neurotransmitter sharpens the senses, leaving them hypersensitive and causes the muscle tension reaction. With tensioned muscles, sickness appears, because digestion can become slower and thus impair the digestive process.

This increase in hormone levels is not established all the time, subsequently the problem that originated externally can be solved, there is a decrease in hormone levels.

Even with the decrease in hormone levels, arteries can be damaged by the frequency and intensity of continued seizures between the amount of hormone production and wear and tear by excessive organic effort.

In this damaging process of the arteries, we still cite cognitive and bone mass weakening. It is important to point out that this cycle suffers constant interference from the environment and how the patient's immune system responds and also his profile and physical conditions.

There are vital needs that make us continue even when we are tired or without a clear expectation of reaching some external object. Unlike what is thought, the demands of life do not come from what we want in the external world, that is, from our material aspirations. This does not cause us melancholy. What demands of us, comes from within.

The demands of life are caught up in our interior and vital needs of existence. The discharge route is related to the principle of pleasure and comes from inside the body. For Freud, in his work Pulsões e Destino das Pulsões (1915), the demands that life demands of us originate primarily from within the body and the corresponding vital needs.

"The pulse will appear to us as a concept situated on the border between the mental and the somatic, as the psychic representative of the stimuli that originate within the organism and reach the mind, as a measure of demand made on the mind to work as a consequence of its connection with the body" (FREUD, 1925, p.127).

The source of the drive is endogenous and is also called the source of the body's interior because of its constancy and its action resulting from the failure of the reflex mechanism to deal with the external factors of desire and how this could be modulated with the internal desire.

The experiences and vicissitudes of our body are mentally inscribed and the neuroses are responses to the inscriptions and demands of work to maintain balance and pacification. It is at the limit between the somatic and the psychic that the pulse is installed.

Freud (1915) states that the pulse is the psychic representative of the stimuli which come from within the body and reach the psyche, as a measure of the work requirement imposed on the psychic as a consequence of his relationship with the body.

The experience of satisfaction is the starting point to deal with the accumulation of energy from somatic needs and psychic activities. This accumulation must be released and it is from the experience of satisfaction that we propose a possible resource for the development of functions that we treat as cognitive: memory, attention, thought, reasoning, problem solving capacity.

This experience is in gradual and experiential maturation, it is not acquired abruptly and fully. Its efficacy lies in constancy and takes place from planning, execution, understanding, storage, and reproduction, actions that can be modified to meet the multiplicity of situations and plural contexts.

## MECHANISM OF SYMPTOM FORMATION: THE MIND

The depression is situated in neurosis, which is part of the psychic instances constituted by the framework of Freudian metapsychology. Neurosis has as its object recalculation, psychosis, foracclusion and perversion to denial. This presupposition presents the paternal position in the relations presented in Freudian theory.

Depression may become a libidinal economy of the new century, in view of the scarce or emptied transfer to the external object, i.e., investment is transferred to the ego, in the service of unrealization.

Apathy, anhedonia and evolution are new forms of perception of an identification that persists in not clenching the thought, distancing the depressive from the human conditions that demand life. This escape from the vicissitudes of daily life makes a mockery of their energies and compromises their libidinal investment in the external object.

This defensive attitude causes paralysis and isolation, not provoking the disposition of excitability and putting in reserve all vital energy that will be inhibited and lost in channelling and self investment.

The World Health Organization (WHO) says that by 2020 depression will be the biggest disabling factor, with the greatest impact until diseases that affect the body with sometimes irreversible damage such as diabetes and angina.

Fleck (2009) considers depression more harmful than angina, arthritis, asthma and diabetes. This veiled way of paralyzing, lowering and emptying the subject's expectations in this 21st century is receiving more and more supporters and efforts for digital media and fabulous relationships of human subjectivation.

The treatment and visibility of this disease alternate between nosological and nosographic, as psychological therapy focused on causes and drug therapy which has the function of regulating and correcting the metabolism of neurotransmitters, i.e. carried out according to the symptoms.

DSM 5 and ICD 10 are descriptive of the articulation of these symptoms to other disorders of the mind, and it is possible to verify the somatization or even the evolution of symptoms from one picture to another. A nosographic description is not the object of psychosomatics, and the knowledge and recognition of signs and symptoms are variable references in the analysis of psychopathological data, which we call data summaries.

Psychoanalytical analysis refutes the idea of a unique and crystallised structure with a verticality in the evolution of the depressive symptom. In the psychic apparatus, one can perceive from the identity of thought to the identity of perception a set of biases and diffusion in the set of signs and symptoms of the depressive process. It is thus known of its internal cause and in these varieties of psychopathological diagnoses, which are fluctuating and intermittent.

The understanding of psychoanalytic theory and the operationalization of all the objects of the seven psychoanalytic schools allow us to affirm that there is no singularity in the depressive process and that this disease is polysymptomatic and distant, zigzagging in dispersed directions. In other words, depression is plural.

As an example, we can say that depression is closely related to neurotic conditions, with psychotics remaining inflexible and unchanged. The signs and symptoms are *ad infinitum* enveloping the subject by the annulment of desire, which becomes meaningless to do simple things in life from taking a bath, watching his film or listening to his favourite music and enjoying his favourite food.

Apathy, lack of mood, lack of hunger and lack of fantasy are part of the symptoms. Depressed people are neurotic and depressed neurotics suffer from living. They only see pain in life and spend their time blaming themselves for not feeling pleasure and for not giving pleasure. This martyrs and corrodes. That's why pain is physical and plurivalent constituting the whole body.

There is an action and reaction in what is expected from the attitudes of a subject in the face of experiential experiences. In these relationships, only desire moves and energises the psychic apparatus. If the blockage in the libidinal investment or the desire becomes scarce, the psychic movement loses its rhythm. To desire something is part of the phenomenon that puts the psychic apparatus to rotate, and in this decrease of pulsional investment, the fuel capable of animating the experiences becomes insufficient and, thus, the wheel stops spinning.

According to Freud (1900), only desire is capable of putting the psychic apparatus into action. The primal experience refers to the reminiscences of the baby's experiences that still persist in our body sculpted in the psychic memory. The prototypes are hunger and the breast, the purpose being the search for satisfaction of this first experience of pleasure.

It is in the encounter between need and other that tension dissipates and pleasure sets in. This other is what makes the role of promoter of this first satisfaction and of realizer of the function of primary care and protection. Mental tracking or facilitation is the repetition of this activity which is satisfied in the whole process of the constitution of contemplation of a perceptive identity, which is also hallucinatory.

Freud treats it as a hallucination, because insistence on the attainment of perceptual identity allows the exhaustive investment in the representation of this primal experience leading to confusion of sense perception, with signs that refer to senses that are not real as regards the temporality of the event, but are in the memory of the subject's recalculated discourse. The imagetic trait left by the experience of satisfaction, it temporalizes in the updating of the saying, which is an action, but does not cease to merge in the hallucinatory act.

The subject does not feel the same pleasure, but is satisfied with the corresponding updating of this experience, and begins to seek redress in the loss. In this game of conformation, there are no winners. The mnemic mark refers to the reminiscences of this support that is inscribed in the memory as an image in the scope of what will be the real of the impossible. This satisfaction is hallucinatory and will bring failure in the pulsional investment, because it results in mental confusion and confrontation between desire and need.

The body will not be satisfied with the image, it desires the material and this movement will not be able to supply this need, resulting in the experience of helplessness. The wear and tear of investment in this imagetic experience that will not be enough to feed the body is unnecessary, but it ruins the investment that would produce the satisfaction of libido.

In the opposite direction of the identity of perception, with the hallucinatory path of desire satisfaction, arises the faculty of thought, which by indirect channel of fulfilment of this experience of satisfaction characterises what is called identity of thought.

Mourning for Freud (Mourning and Melancholy, Freud, 1917) is a cause of relative impoverishment of the self and inhibition of the mechanism of topographic balance, which feeds only one of the instances in the topic. Reactions to loss are of an ideal or material nature. Regarding melancholy, we can associate the various biases that are traversed in the phenomenological Freudian description of the mourning process.

In this journey, there is the impoverishment of the self weakened by the lost object, which, when it is disfigured, is depersonalized. It is important to confirm that from this point of view, the psychotic structure is very similar to the symptoms of melancholy, even though it is a very delicate subject, we start here to use the Freudian line of clinical reasoning of approximation of melancholy with psychosis.

The most complex thing in the process of mourning and melancholy is to understand that the lost object does not bring pain, but rather pincers the process of mourning for the replacement of this object, without the awareness of the identity of thought. For Freud, the painful thing is not the loss of the object, but the hard work of mourning and its hypersensation of attachment to the representation of the lost object. In this case, it is the pain of connection that demands hyperinvestment and not the pain of separation, what hurts is not separating but becoming more and more attached.

We have launched the apparent and decisive distinction for the clinic of depression in the elementary concepts between loss and fault. The defence is in a constant narcissistic relationship for overcoming the depressive process and consequent substitution, as the propelling element of the healing process. In the lack, we have what is the propelling motor of the desire for life and in the loss the incursion into the perceptive identity of connection to the lost object. As well as the antidote to loss, there is only the substitutive representation of lack.

## *CASE* AND ILLUSTRATIVE MEDICAL HISTORY

Clinical follow-up activities refer to preventive and intervention actions, with psychopathological diagnosis, of signs and symptoms in evolution. This topic is initiated with the presentation of a clinical history fragment described by Bottura Jr (2009, p. 87), one of the most useful disseminators of psychosomatics in Brazil, President of the Brazilian Association of Psychosomatic Medicine - National.

### *Case 01*

*The report had been made following a temporal order. It highlights the situation experienced by the newly graduated physician Olimpio, who even though he had an intense and dynamic professional life, would have gone to the bank to renew a loan that he had been unable to repay.*

*(...)*

*In the brief moment he was on the bench, Olimpio noticed the entrance of another doctor who, when addressing the manager, receives the guidance to also sit in the small waiting room. Olimpio thought: "What a well-dressed, elegant doctor he is going to deposit", and was intimidated in the chair.*

*(...)*

*Olimpio was most frightened when he realized that besides everything he was still wearing the changed shoes, although white and many alike, they were of different pairs.*

*(...)*

*"The other doctor pulled conversation, and then Olimpio could no longer be incognito. After a few minutes of chatting, the other started to complain about the situation, saying that he was there to extend a payment. At that moment, our insecure and shaken Olimpio breathed again and thought: 'Good, I'm not the only one!', but he had not taken his foot off the table. "*

*(...)*

*Olimpio left the bank relieved, then renewed the loan. However, he thought everyone was looking at his feet with their shoes changed. The only way to go unnoticed was to walk faster.*

**DISCUSSION**

Internal dialogues refer to *every action of the human being, each movement, consists in the representation of an internal dialogue. (BOTTURE, 2009, p.69).* For these internal dialogues to be in balance, it is indispensable that self-knowledge, self-evaluation, and the identification of emotions and feelings allow for an operationalization of these feelings and also their expression.

Evolution requires us to be constantly balanced. These processes of emptying and filling are intensely related to the concepts of ideal of perception and thought. In this orientation, it is from the stressful experiences that we come to understand, through the discomforts and vicissitudes, the experiences of satisfaction.

The worst way to deal with these relations of balance and imbalance is to invest libidinally in misguided defences. The undue reaction to the event or the stressful situation is that it provokes a series of responses that trigger other negative effects and biases.

CLINICAL DEVICES

| MODERNITY<br>FIRST CLINIC | | |
|---|---|---|
| **1953 – 1970**<br>**Lacan's First Clinic** | **Criticism of analyst mirroring** | **Classic**<br>**Freudism** |
| 1. Paternity | Father/parent guidance | Oedipus Complex |
| 2. Jerarquization | Hierarchy/submission | Superego |
| 3. Intercommunication | Dialogue/face-to-face | Therapeutic alliance |
| 4. Streamlining | Anti-syncretic/reason reasoning | Other |
| 5. Universalization | Established truth / fact | Supposed to know |
| 6. Inertization | Static/imobile | Resistance |
| 7. Analyticity | Evaluation/analysis | Hard symptom |
| 8. Training | Training | Methodology |
| 9 Verticalism | Authority/empty | Specularity |
| 10. Tribulation | Difficulty/adversity | Repression |

**Source: School of Health in Psychosomatic Medicine**

| WORLDWIDE<br>SECOND CLINIC | | |
|---|---|---|
| **1970 – 1981**<br>**Second Lacan Clinic** | **Criticism of analyst mirroring** | **Lacanism** |
| 1. Change | Alterity | Collective calculation |
| 2. Dissipation | Reversibility | Radical differences |
| 3. Intradiscourse | Internalisation | Articulated monologues |
| 4. Accessibility | Sharing | Resessoar |
| 5. Flexibility | Mobility | Certainty |
| 6. Connectivity | Relational | Interactive |
| 7. Empatibility | Altruism | Responsibility |
| 8. Likelihood | Vicissitudes | Experiences |
| 9 Horizontalism | Dimensionality | Horizontal order |
| 10. Iteration | Intelligence | Opportunity |

**Source: School of Health in Psychosomatic Medicine**

| MEANINGS AND RESIGNATIONS PSYCHOSOCIAL | | |
| --- | --- | --- |
| **Experiences Exhausting/ Satisfaction** | **Devices** | **Emotions and Feelings** |
| **1.** Behaviour manifested | Selves: self grandiose exhibitionist/spe cular and self tripolar | Perception of real or imaginary danger (fear) / Psychic manifestation as a response to emotional discomfort as a response to trauma. |
| **2.** Meaning and resignified | Psychic elaboration/Prim ary Narcissism/Mirro r Radio/Object a. | Self-evaluation and self-knowledge; ideal of perception and ideal of thought; recognition of image; lack and crossing of anguish by desire. |
| **3.** Reminiscenc es and memorable meanings | Clinical management: transfer, pulse, unconscious and repetition. | Perpetual and stressful cyclic repetition. Negative reaction as an inadequate defence to the stressful and stressful experience/phobia and difficulty in resuming simple activities. |
| **4.** Grief and melancholy | Quaternary structure/desire (lack) /object a. | Fear, anger and sadness and their respective feelings. (Anguish, stress, anxiety, loneliness and insecurity). |
| **5.** Result | Primary narcissism, Objective love, Oedipus Complex, In the Name of the Father, Castration. | Resumption of infantile feelings and emotions inherent in infantile life and its compositions of psychic elaboration. |
| **6.** Image Representati ons | Borromean/real node, symbolic and imaginary. | Meanings consisting of meanings. Ideals of perception and their ideological or symbolic representations. |

**Source: School of Health in Psychosomatic Medicine**

The conception of psychosomatics relates to the three articulated and dynamic pillars (mind, body and social relationships), because it is understood by social interaction and even if the concept is developed to encompass the most distinct areas of human and technological knowledge, it can be said that the indissociability of mind, body and social relationships is in human nature. It is in the concatenated representation between Psychogenic, Medical Psychology and Medical Anthropology that the primordial elements of these psychosomatic currents are highlighted.

Transferencial and contratransferencial analysis in a biopsychosocial scenario in psychosomatic medicine pincers the treatment of the disease as a pathological structure, however the psychic dimension of the patient must be integrated. Psychosomatics had its beginning in the 1950s, and it is relevant to highlight the mobilization of medical professionals who were caudatários of studies in Psychoanalysis and lived in the cities of São Paulo and Rio de Janeiro.

It is important to stress that psychosomatics is not the discovery of a new path in the clinical area but only the resumption of a discussion among health professionals who had in their practice a relational *modus operandi* between the ideal of body and soul in the studies that were oriented towards the search for cure and the minimization of eminently pathological symptoms and somatic structure.

The affirmation that the most consolidated directive of Psychosomatics is a reorganization in the way of seeing the pathology that affects the organism and of the therapeutic action focused on the sick subject is the root of a lens of the clinic centered on man as a subject constituted by history, its social, anthropological, philosophical and dialectic development.

The singular precept of psychosomatics is based on the focus of the subject who has an illness and its biopsychosocial nature and not on the biologicism of the illness that affects the subject. It can be said that Psychosomatics would be a new version of the investigation of the pathology, of the way of analysing the person who has this pathology and its relation with the therapy used in the treatment.

The pragmatic use of psychoanalysis in psychosomatics has been due to the irrefutable contribution of including free association, as an act of speaking about what one feels and what bothers the patient in the clinical scene and how the symbolic (word) could denote a new perspective to pathogenesis.

This approach has attributed to oneiric processes, fantasies, faulty acts and impulses, being the necessary reception of the constitution of senses of the subject's daily life. The illness would no longer be the memorable one of meanings. It would be this assertion the role of light, shadow and penumbra in an analysis of the principle of rectilinear propagation of light in its metaphorization by the healing process.

# PSYCHOANALYSIS AND PSYCHOMOTRICITY

The understanding of the dynamic nature of the symptom in a psychoanalytic lens of cultural matrix goes through a historical incursion, as the constitution of the subject affected by the symbolic, the history, the real of the language. Destutt of Tracy (1801), in defining ideology as the relationship of man with the environment, impregnated the term with a positive idea, and then Bonaparte and Marx and Engels tried to reverse this logic. Althusser, Pêcheux, Foucault and Ricoeur analyzed the discourse under a matrix and catalytic lens, contributing to this tessitura of interconnected elements tinged by the understanding that extrapolates a restricted thought of masking reality. It is impossible to escape from ideology, because it constitutes us; it operates for us and over us.

"Thus considered, ideology is not an occult, but a function of the necessary relationship between language and the world" (ORLANDI, 1999, p.47).

In speaking of Psychoanalysis, such a study is immediately related to Freud, since it is on it that all the precepts referenced by the study of the unconscious are based. According to him, the theories of sexuality and the unconscious mind are the basis of every psychoanalytic study.

In its genesis, the understanding, understanding and applicability of the theory of the human psyche are observed in this universe: its establishing source, form of action, and constitution. Studies on the process of appropriation of knowledge and its application in the social world are closely related to the assumptions of psychoanalytic theory.

Psychoanalysis is thus a theory which has as its principle the understanding that behaviour and feelings are governed by unconscious desires, and that mainly cases of neurosis and psychosis are treated by this therapeutic method devised by S. Freud. In this sense, the unconscious contents of words, actions and imaginary productions of an individual are treated by the psychoanalyst's analysis, based on free associations and transference, the psychoanalytic lens. It emerges from this that, since it is a clinical and theoretical field of investigation of the human **psyche,** independent of psychology, it has its origin in medicine, a theory developed by this psychoanalyst.

The theory of psychoanalysis contributes greatly to the understanding of the constitution of the subject. It does not become pertinent, after Freud, to analyse childhood in a restricted way, as a bridge marked by organic development. We are beings affected by the symbolic and through it we become agents of our history, since we are not biologically created but historically formed.

Michel Pêcheux (1938-1983) presents a theory which is based on the conception materialised in ideology and of how ideology manifests itself. The discourse for Pêcheux is the space that derives from the relationship between language and ideology, as an effect of senses. Thus, the explanation of the mechanisms of historical determination of the processes of meaning is the major objective of the discourse analyst and it is by the analysis of the discursive functioning that this is achieved.

It is important to highlight the influences of Althusser and Canguilhem in Pêcheux's works, because from the theoretical contributions of these authors, a transformation in the practice of the human and social sciences was proposed, through an analysis of the philosophy of empirical knowledge and the history of epistemology.

The question involving the political and the symbolic is seen as a space for confrontation, but it is from this idea of confrontation that questions are first of all brought to Linguistics about excluded exteriority and, in this orientation, also questions the Social Sciences about the transparency of language, the foundation of the evidence on which these Sciences are conceived.

A system subject to ambiguity, this is how Pêcheux considers discursiveness. The deutomatisation of language is the fluid nature observed by the autonomy instituted by the relations of metaphor (transference). Literality is no longer the connecting support where words seek meaning. Meaning is always sought in the other, that is, in a symbolic *locus*, founded on movement because it is historical.

Pêcheux has its rhizome constituted by Linguistics, Marxism and Psychoanalysis, but it does not conform to their postulates and questions them about language, history and subject. For Lacan, the signifier is expressed through desire. Thus, one can perceive an immediate relationship with the unconscious, immediate but constant. We are desiring beings, then, we are signifiers; the constituted speech itself.

In this orientation, Sausurian theory defines language as a system of signs, while language for Jacques Lacan is conceptualized as a structure that exists prior to the subject's entrance at the moment of his mental development. S. Freud talks about speech:

The expression 'speech' should be understood not only as meaning the expression of thought in words, but including the language of gestures and all other methods, such as writing, through which mental activity can be expressed (FREUD, 1974, p. 211).

The primacy of the signifier (acoustic image) over the meaning (concept) is an indispensable precept for the understanding of the founding elements of Psychoanalysis, with regard to the object of this science. This theoretical shift is crucial for the conception of a subject in the field of the symbolic, that is, the very confirmation of the idea of the unconscious structured as language.

The unconscious is not a species defined in psychic reality by the circle of what does not have the attribute (or virtue) of consciousness" (LACAN, 1966, p. 830).

The unconscious consists of the repressed materials.

"The unconscious is not losing one's memory; it is not remembering what one knows (LACAN, 2001, p. 333).

For Lacan (1956), it is in systemic approaches to structure that unconscious desire is organised by means of language through the symbolic. It is in this field of language that the subject constitutes himself in relation to the other. In this orientation, the symbolic is perceived as an action of *decentralisation* introduced by the notion of the unconscious, of Freudian psychoanalysis.

The symbols envelop the life of man in such a total net that they bring together, before he comes into the world, those who will engender him "*by bone and flesh*"; who bring at his birth, with the gifts of the stars, if not the gifts of the fairies, the design of his destiny (LACAN, 1966, p. 279).

For Lacan (1972), the three conceptual categories symbolic, imaginary and real refer to the symbolic which is the space which contemplates language. It is in this interstice that the subject and the law and order, which are called Other, are related. The subject is circumscribed in the instance of the conscious and unconscious. Thus it can be affirmed that the unconscious has its manifestation in language and this is represented in the psychoanalytic clinic by means of free association, the faulty act, the chistes, the dreams and the symptoms.

Lacan (1998) describes language as symbolic, since it is through it that the system of representations, based on signifiers, determines the subject in its revelation.

It is through this symbolic system that the subject refers to himself by using language (ROUDINESCO; PLON, 1998).

In the notional act of subject, for Lacan, the subject ceases to be, becoming the subject of the unconscious. History plays a fundamental role in this Interchange.

The Lacanian subject finds existence at a crossroads where a work on the letter and the signifier and a decentralized position of the self in relation to the process of speech intersect. These two (relatively) independent axes indirectly draw a place whose register of functioning is henceforth ensured by the canonical definition according to which the signifier represents the subject to another.

## PSYCHOANALYSIS AND THEORIES: PRACTICES AND IDEOLOGY OF THE OCCULT

The proposal is to present an approach of Psychoanalysis articulated to linguistic theories and new codes and technologies and social media, in a model of convergence with connection between subjects in a society of integration and high dimension of information exchange, emphasizing the understanding/apprehension of multiple meanings, according to the socio-economic-cultural-historical-political situation of the region.

In the interrelationship between psychoanalytical knowledge and integrated and participatory educational practice in this collaborative and convergent society, it is necessary to present Freud's essential concepts: unconsciousness, drive, sexuality, aggressiveness, defense mechanisms and the phases of personality development, as well as their updating for the other seven schools of psychoanalysis.

In this guideline, the reading of Freud's work by Lacan and revisited by him is indispensable for the social and cultural understanding of psychoanalysis, especially with regard to the constitution of the subject by the other and by speech, in its object of fault.

Winnicott (1975), a paediatrician and psychoanalyst, was born into a thriving family in Plymouth, Great Britain, on April 7, 1896, and developed a model of understanding small children in their relationship of dependence on a "good motherhood" for the construction of a cultural, social and political identity based on virtues based on the scope of morality, ethics and citizenship.

Thus, the potential to be developed in children is interconnected to this symbolic moment which is maternal influence (and in the meantime includes the paternal one) in the construction of this great Other with the force of ideological determination of interpellation and crossing. The subject is challenged by this ideology and put in relation with history.

The affective bonds in the different phases of the child's development and their respective consequences in the course of the life of this subject of wills and desires are the object of study of Pichon-Riviére. The social relationships that are built up in the various social microcosms (school, church, parties, groups, etc.) substantiate or reject the concepts incorporated by family practices.

It is in these multifaceted spaces of identity formation and of the symbolic and imaginary that true interpersonal relationships are exchanged. The educational practice in the social reality of the subject in a society of convergence and collaboration is created, deconstructed and reconstructed from the dialectical processes in constant movement.

This is a dynamic that does not dispense with any approach and interconnects with the most distinct *psycho-pedagogical and cultural doings*, not limited to deterministic, linear theories and areas of exclusionary and superficial thinking of a purely positivist basis.

The hypnotic method had been abandoned as soon as the free association method emerged. The discovery of speech as cathartic is able to recall the traumatic experiences and was the cause for the abandonment of hypnosis and, also, because it was invasive of personality, it would not be indicated to all patients.

Hypnosis would thus gradually become ineffective and a method would have to be created that was not restricted to a particular public and could be used without reservation. The method of free association is basically the method of speech, at which point the patient talks about what he or she wants and in what way. The idea is that unconscious contents become conscious due to associations, through words.

# STAGES OF A PSYCHOPATHOLOGICAL PSYCHOANALYTICAL RESEARCH

Ordination in the psychopathological field is essential to use the elements that would function as data summaries.

The first key is composed of descriptive psychopathology, its object being the form of the symptom, establishing the description of the psychic alterations. The content of these alterations is the focus of dynamic psychopathology, the stressful experiences and their expressions. They are the affections, fears, disillusionment of people in their specificity; this is not always possible to be described or systematized.

The second key is a pole called medical psychopathology, thus relating the studies linked to the assertive of brain malfunctioning. This orientation sees a dysfunction, i.e. poor regulation in the organ or system. On the other hand, existential psychopathology sees the singularity, the specificity and the unique way of analysing the being and of understanding the particular nuances of being, in the elementary dimension the historical questions of a symbolic field with meanings and resignifications are based. It can be said, then, that being is the conjunction of all the singularly elementary experiences of a subject who acts in his history and intervenes dynamically in the formations and transformations of his psychic reality.

In key three, the opposition between the objects of analysis of behavioural and psychoanalytical psychopathology highlights a consideration of man as a set of possible observable and measurable behaviours to be regulated. This cognitive aspect is possibly verified and amenable to modelling, being of order and conscious formation.

Psychoanalytical psychopathology presents a determination of the subject through conflicts and unconscious desires. It sees man as a desirous being always clinging to the order of the symbolic. It is in the psyche that affections dominate and from the expressions of conflicts, inherent basically in the traumatic contents of infantile life, emerge as somatological symptoms.

The fourth key is the one containing the operational-pragmatic psychopathology that is involved in the function of serving as a systematic scope for the constitution of the Diagnostic and Statistical Manual of Mental Disorders-DSM 5 and other manuals, ICD - International Statistical Classification of Diseases and Problems Related to Health and CIF - International Classification of Functionality, Disability and Health. In contrast, fundamental psychopathology refers to the foundation of each psychopathological definition.

It is the French psychoanalyst Pierre Fédida who proposes an idea of the meaning of the symptom as passion and suffering. It is the *pathos*! The intrinsic relationship of the unsustainable lightness of being involved in a link of passion and passivity before the motility of human relationships.

Key number five is the dimensional psychopathology which predicts the gradual evolution of signs, symptoms and disorders. An example of this analysis would be the autistic spectrum, which analyses as rain guard and the evolutionary relationships of signs and symptoms, with sometimes comorbid characteristics.

This guidance is best suited to an up-to-date clinical context of transdisciplinary clinical work. The segmentation and structuring and analysis of mental disorders in an individualized manner as a nosological entity is the hallmark of categorical psychopathology. This type of psychopathology requires a unitary diagnostic identification and belongs to a biologically demarcated field.

The sixth and last key belongs to two distinct types of psychopathology: sociocultural and biological. The first analyses and treats the symptom as socially and culturally constituted, both symbolic and historical. It is in the cultural matrix that all the elements that will guide to what is normal and what is pathological are based, which would then be socially accepted by a certain community.

The focus on the neurophysiology of mental disorder is the work of biological psychopathology, i.e. brain and neurochemical aspects. The basis would then be the alteration of neural functioning and brain constitution mechanisms.

Thus, the evaluation, for the selection of psychopathology, be it of any nature, is related to the fact of carrying out an analysis in a specific dimension, that is, it can make use of logical-mathematical reasoning, verbal-linguistic orientation, intrapersonal or interpersonal nature, cultural manifestation, manifesto, personality relations and cognitive and intelligence components.

This analysis can be of values, with quantitative and cutaneous tangency, being by calculations and guided by mathematics in an objective way subsidizing itself of human characteristics or behaviour or psychic nature. What is confirmed is that the concatenation is in the link with the valuation of the object of value with determination given by the one who evaluates and makes his or her analyst lens valid. This analyst systematises the knowledge related to the steps of valuation, the forms and guidelines of analysis, with a defined scope and a technique of quantitative or qualitative analysis.

Analytical procedures and methods, whether they are behavioural or objective in their historical-constitutive relationship, are circumscribed in the application of analytical instruments and techniques. Then, it can be said that they emerge from the need to understand human behavioural phenomena and in the prediction, interpretation and explanation of these phenomena.

There is no disdain for empirical, philosophical and theological knowledge, but it is in observable, validated, reproducible knowledge, which is scientific, that we cling to any kind of analysis in the field of human evaluation, it takes place in science and through methodology.

This series of procedures and methods of analysis of what the evaluation is about has in the scientificity its more specific and effective nature and it is in the sessions, in the instruments and techniques of evaluation that the conditions of the methods and techniques of operational applicability of the evaluation instrument are related.

It is always important to base the evaluation on an operative contextualisation component, because the context in which the evaluation is inserted is fertile soil of assertiveness and guarantee of reliability. The clinic operates in its assertiveness, the misunderstanding is of the order of who practices it.

The psychoanalytical constructs to be investigated are derived from instances of psychic studies and their respective approaches, psychoanalytical, behavioural, systemic and others. The knowledge and recognition of these lines enables the interrelated probability of articulation and complementarity, in a care that is multiprofessional, because psychoanalysis is thus of constitution.

The theoretical basis refers to the precise and objective knowledge of the phenomena to be evaluated, investigating in an operational way the psychopathological components of signs, symptoms, disorders and illnesses, knowing that the knowledge of signs and symptoms enables a psychopathological diagnosis of an investigative nature.

It is in the reference of the theoretical, technical, methodological and instrumental/scientific process that the whole evaluation process must be based, being at the moment of data collection that the tools and techniques planned for the evaluation are handled.

Upon completion of the evaluation process, decisions and strategies are measured and result in the operationalization of actions and attitudes, as well as the planning of interventions during the evaluation process. This is the basis for the preparation of the report, which will be written according to the specificity of the previous items: multiprofessional report, declaration, attestation and opinion, which are types of reports resulting from the evaluation.


## THE QUATERNARY STRUCTURE IN PSYCHOANALYTIC PSYCHOPATHOLOGY

Below are possible steps for the elaboration of an analysis in psychoanalytical psychopathology:

1.  Free association/healing process
2.  Demand/cure process
3.  Dimensioning and resizing the symptom
4.  Transfer and Contratransfer

The coding device is capable of measuring these risks and the probability of index and reference of the symptom addressed in the subject. Evaluation of any kind is related to the fact that an analysis is carried out in a specific dimension.

Thus, this analysis can be valued and interrelated, but always subjective. The discussion about the new unconscious enables a systematic organization of the clinical devices of psychoanalysis.

The basis of the purposes of psychoanalytical evaluation guides the global and specific objectives of the work of psychopathological evaluation and humanized accompaniment of a subject made up of history and touched by the symbolic, thus adapting the characteristics of the instruments and techniques to the clinical devices of schools of thought and their respective objects.

When we think of free association as a method used by Saint Freud, in order to make the analysis speak what came to his mind, we return to the early days of Freud's substitution of hypnosis as a resource for the treatment of hysteria, in the first studies on this treatise. The free association of ideas is the promising path towards the access to the unconscious, as it was referred to in a *regimen*.

The dimensioning and resizing of the symptom is a binary activity, an exercise in the psychoanalytical *setting* that refers to the analyst and analyzing. The analyst dimensions his symptom by means of the senses, by the way in which he dispenses with a series of events at the core of his existence. He has contact with his griefs and dimensions them according to his egóic property of social representation.

Redimensioning is a brief task for the analyst who perceives the biases and condensations of his fantasy. It is not just any fabrication; it is a ritual of elements, acts and facts that relate in a dynamic and decipherable way, from the point of view of interpretation. Return to the genesis of the object of recalculation. To proceed in a legitimate way to the call of the real.

The desire of the analyst based on his perceptions, comparisons and sublimations are presented in the demand offered to the analyst. In the demand, one finds what is contained in his libidinal request to the analyst. The energy already drained and the product of the losses reveal when analysing a sense crystallised and stuck to the social.

The transfer and contract transfer are articulated for the operationalization of demand in the psychoanalytical *setting*. The possibility of fruition without the intervention of repression in the clinic takes place in a manner elaborated by the analyst and the empathy that results from the commitment to this relationship, the commitment coming from the analyst, which is the contra-transference produces the effect of an analytical procedure. The relationships that take place in the psychoanalytic clinic between analyst and analyst in the process of transference and countertransference.

The healing process is the answer to psychoanalytic treatment, as we are split, cleaved and incomplete subjects. The healing process is the understanding of this lack and their commitment to present their experiences, to the new, to the tense situations that will make them patients in psychic treatment during their whole neurotic existence.

## EDUCATION AND PSYCHOMOTRICITY

ADHD (Attention Deficit Disorder, with Hyperactivity, Impulsivity and Inattention) is characterized by a dysfunction in the prefrontal cortex and has as its symptoms impulsivity, inattention disorders, loss of control of emotions, difficulty in planning, developing strategies and hyperactivity, with hyperkinesia. According to ARRUDA (2019), 912,000 Brazilian children between 5 and 12 years of age are affected by ADHD symptoms, an estimated 3.3% of the child population, as presented by IBGE. Children with ADHD have seven times greater risk of suffering domestic accidents and nine times greater chance of being hospitalized for bruises and fractures, and in adult life there is also a greater risk of difficulty in maintaining personal relationships and a greater possibility of developing suicidal ideation.

Although there are indications for ADHD treatment with amphetamines and stimulants (Arruda, 2019), it is important to highlight the role of cognitive components in frontal "maturation" and the significant contribution of psychotherapies and cognitive-behavioral activity. In this orientation, physical activities, i.e. the development of motor activities, play a fundamental role in all the psychic aspects of these children and adolescents in the school phase.

The diagnosis should take into account various criteria, both educational, social, family and clinical. This clinical condition is very common, so it affects a significant portion of the child population, about 5%, and these symptoms, if not treated, will persist in adult life, manifesting as agitation, impulsiveness and inattention.

The ADHD Research Center for Latin America participated in its research at the Instituto D'Or de Pesquisa e Ensino, in Rio de Janeiro, with representation of Dr. Paulo Mattos.

This research included more than 3,000 people, ADHD patients and healthy individuals, between 4 and 63 years of age, who underwent structural neuroimaging by MRI. A posteriori, each region of the brain was evaluated. This protocol can present a comparison of brain structures between individuals with and without the disorder.

The result of the research was very important for the evidence that the structures of ADHD patients such as hippocampus, accumbens nucleus and tonsils are smaller, thus knowing that they are responsible for motivation and regulation of emotions, as well as the so-called reward system. When it is perceived that in adults these changes are less significant, we have proof that this disorder is related to the delayed maturation of brain regions that regulate emotions and have as audience mainly children.

It is important to point out the difference between Attention Deficit Disorder, of the inattentive type and the hyperactive type, and the impulsive type must also receive specific and directed care. The act of making careless mistakes, difficulty in keeping the attention directive and operative, following instructions, organizing tasks and forgetting, is related to inattention.

The hyperactive and combined type presents the behaviour of continuous movement, going out of place to move voluntarily, running or climbing, talking excessively. The symptoms of inattention are most commonly perceived and evidenced in female children. It is important to point out that current literature no longer admits a visible epidemiological distinction between boys and girls when the subject is ADHD.

ADHD is a neurodevelopmental disorder that has current severity specification, according to the Diagnostic and Statistical Manual of Mental Disorders - DSM 5, of the *American Psychiatric Association - APA*: 1. Light, with few symptoms, if any, are present beyond those needed to make the diagnosis, criteria met in six (6) months. Other specifications refer to the social, academic or professional life of the patient. 2. Moderate, symptoms or functional damage between "mild" and "severe" are present. 3. severe, many symptoms other than those necessary to make the diagnosis are present, or the symptoms may result in severe impairment.

According to data presented by Sheftall *et al.*, (2016), ADHD is the most diagnosed neurodevelopmental disorder when studying cases of suicide in children under 12 years of age. Research of this nature points to the need to discuss the importance of disorders that are presented in people who do not yet have their brain regions biologically developed (hypothalamus and amygdala as opposed to the prefrontal cortex). The research done by the American Journal Pediatrics in 17 US states, between the years 2012 and 2013 brought a significant understanding of the relationship between the disorder and suicide deaths.

The sample was 87 children between 5 and 11 years and 606 pre-adolescents between 12 and 14 years. The procedure was comparative, with one third of each group presenting a type of mental disorder. In the case of children, diagnosed with ADHD, hyperactivity or impulsiveness, making up 1/3 and in the case of pre-adolescents, 2/3 with symptoms of depression and dysthymia.

The author of the study, Arielle H. Sheftall, Ph.D., at Nationwide Children's Hospital in Columbus, Ohio, said that in the case of pre-adolescent suicides there was a general pattern of stressful experiences (friends, family, school and affective and social relationships) but those with some kind of mental disorder were more often diagnosed with ADHD.

Other important data relating to this alarming suicide and ADHD situation have been presented by The National Resource Center on ADHD (CHADD). BARBARESI (2013) presented results on his ADHD studies based on clinical records of 5,718 adults and found that 8% of the 367 adults who had ADHD in childhood committed suicide, with only 1% of the 4,946 adults without ADHD committing it (Chad.org).

BARKLEY (2008) indicated that adults with ADHD histories are twice as likely to consider or attempt suicide at age 21. A study by the National Comorbidity Replication Survey (NCS-R) confirmed that of 365 adults with current ADHD, 16% had attempted suicide. According to Agosti (2011), even though the prediction factor of attempted suicide was not confirmed, having one or more disorders increased the risk by 4-12 times. (Chad.org).

HINSHAW (2012) after a 10-year prospective study of girls with ADHD in early adulthood found that of 93 girls with combined ADHD, 22 percent attempted suicide compared with the inattentive type, 8 percent, and 6 percent of 88 girls with no history of ADHD. These figures are relevant to the misconception that the focus on males is exclusive when it comes to identification, diagnosis, intervention and treatment of ADHD.

Studies relating to education and psychomotricity have extrapolated the eminently cognitive difficulties of the classroom in reading, writing and calculating. The object of psychomotricity in education is oriented from the processes of teaching and human learning (cognitive, emotional and motor), with the operationalization of knowledge and protagonism in social interventions, thus actively participating in the construction of society. The family, which is the *mother* cell of society, is the driving force and driving point of this relationship. Therefore, it is in the inseparable relationship between cognitive, emotional and motor that the studies of articulation between education and psychomotricity are based.

The school is the social microcosm that proposes the regulatory exercise of the organization of society. It is from there that social norms and rules emanate from what is or is not allowed, from the very first years of children's lives, and psycho-pedagogy thus studies these evolving patterns of what is common, normal and pathological.

It is in the response to the inseparable relationships between education, culture and society and the influence of the environment in which we live and develop that, fundamentally, psychomotricity comprises human action in the social organisation of children, young people and adults with interaction and learning difficulties. Effective action goes beyond exercises and motor activities to insert the subject, which is made up of history and touched by the symbolic, in the social universe, of psychosomatic relationships between mind, body and social relationships.

# BIBLIOGRAPHICAL REFERENCES

American Psychiatry Association. *Diagnostic and Statistical Manual of Mental disorders - DSM-5.* 5th.ed. Washington: American Psychiatric Association, 2013.

JUNIOR BOTTURE, Wimer. Silent aggressions: the communication contagion/Wimer Bottura Júnior - 3rd Edition - São Paulo: Literary Republic, 2009.

FOUCAULT, M. *Microfisica of power.* Rio de Janeiro: Grail, 1979.

______. *The birth of the clinic.* Rio de Janeiro: Forensic, 2001.

______. *The abnormals: course at the Collège de France.* São Paulo: Martins Fontes, 2001

FREUD, S. *Totem and taboo.* Rio de Janeiro: Imago, 1987. v.13.

______. *The unease in civilization.* Saint Paul: Imago, 1992. v.21

______. *On the psychopathology of daily life.* Rio de Janeiro: Imago, 1996. v.6.

______. *Freud's psychoanalytical method.* Rio de Janeiro: Imago, 1996. v.7.

______. *The dynamics of the transfer.* Rio de Janeiro: Imago, 1996. v.12.

______. *Recall, repeat and elaborate.* Rio de Janeiro: Imago, 1996. v.12.

______. *Comments on transference love.* Rio de Janeiro: Imago, 1996. v.12.

______. *On narcissism: an introduction.* Rio de Janeiro: Imago, 1996. v.14.

______. *On transitority.* Rio de Janeiro: Imago, 1996. v.14.

______. *The instincts and their vicissitudes.* Rio de Janeiro: Imago, 1996. v.14.

______. Grief *and melancholy.* Rio de Janeiro: Imago, 1996. v.14.

______. *The "stranger".* Rio de Janeiro: Imago, 1996. v.17.

______. *Group psychology and ego analysis.* Rio de Janeiro: Imago, 1996. v.18.

______. *The ego and the id.* Rio de Janeiro: Imago, 1996. v.19.

______. *Neurosis and psychosis.* Rio de Janeiro: Imago, 1996. v.19.

______. *Inhibitions, symptoms and distress.* Rio de Janeiro: Imago, 1996. v.20.

______. *The humor.* Rio de Janeiro: Imago, 1996. v.21.

______. *Beyond the pleasure principle.* Rio de Janeiro: Imago, 1998.

LEAR, K. (2004). *Help Us Learn: A Self-Paced Training Program for ABA.* (2ED). Toronto. Taken from: http://www. autism. psychology-science. com. br/wp-content/uploads/2012/07/Autism-help us learn. pdf

MELO-SON, Julio de. Psychosomatics today/Julio de Mello-Filho [et al.] - 2 - Porto Alegre: Artmed, 2010.

World Health Organization-WHO. *International Classification of Diseases and Health Related Problems. ICD-l0.* 8 São Paulo: EDUSP, 2000. 119p.

C. Psychopathology Psychoanalytic: the study of man by the determination of his desires and unconscious conflicts. New Academic Editions (*International Book Market Service Ltd., member of OmniScriptum Publishing Group*), Mauritius, 2020.

SILVA, Maria Cecília A. e. **Psycho-pedagogy**: in search of a theoretical foundation. Rio de Janeiro: Nova Fronteira, 1998.

VISCA, Jorge. **Psycho-pedagogical clinic**: convergent epistemology. São José dos Campos: Pulso Editorial, 2010.

WEISS, M.L.L. **Overcoming school learning difficulties**. Rio de Janeiro: Wak Editora, 2009.

WEISS, Maria L. **Clinical psycho-pedagogy**: a diagnostic view of learning problems. Rio de Janeiro: DP&A, 2006.

# ANNEXES - Activities - Curriculum

| Development of Motor/Power Skills | | | |
|---|---|---|---|
| **Visual contact** | | | |
| Item | Behaviour | Response | As a result |
| 1 | | | |
| 2 | | | |
| 3 | | | |
| 4 | | | |
| 5 | | | |
| 6 | | | |
| 7 | | | |
| 8 | | | |
| 9 | | | |
| 10 | | | |

| Development of Motor/Power Skills | | | |
|---|---|---|---|
| **Imitation** | | | |
| Item | Behaviour | Response | As a result |
| 1 | | | |
| 2 | | | |
| 3 | | | |
| 4 | | | |
| 5 | | | |
| 6 | | | |
| 7 | | | |
| 8 | | | |
| 9 | | | |
| 10 | | | |

| Development of Motor/Power Skills | | | |
|---|---|---|---|
| **Receptive Language** | | | |
| Item | Behaviour | Response | As a result |
| 1 | | | |
| 2 | | | |
| 3 | | | |
| 4 | | | |
| 5 | | | |
| 6 | | | |
| 7 | | | |
| 8 | | | |
| 9 | | | |
| 10 | | | |

| Motor/psychomotor Skills Development | | | |
| Expressive Language | | | |
| Item | Behaviour | Response | As a result |
|---|---|---|---|
| 1 | | | |
| 2 | | | |
| 3 | | | |
| 4 | | | |
| 5 | | | |
| 6 | | | |
| 7 | | | |
| 8 | | | |
| 9 | | | |
| 10 | | | |

| Development of Motor/Power Skills | | | |
| Alternative Communication | | | |
| Item | Behaviour | Response | As a result |
|---|---|---|---|
| 1 | | | |
| 2 | | | |
| 3 | | | |
| 4 | | | |
| 5 | | | |
| 6 | | | |
| 7 | | | |
| 8 | | | |
| 9 | | | |
| 10 | | | |

| Development of Motor/Power Skills | | | |
| Inhibitory Control | | | |
| Item | Behaviour | Response | As a result |
|---|---|---|---|
| 1 | | | |
| 2 | | | |
| 3 | | | |
| 4 | | | |
| 5 | | | |
| 6 | | | |
| 7 | | | |
| 8 | | | |
| 9 | | | |
| 10 | | | |

| Development of Motor/Power Skills | | | |
|---|---|---|---|
| **Shared Attention** | | | |
| Item | Behaviour | Response | As a result |
| 1 | | | |
| 2 | | | |
| 3 | | | |
| 4 | | | |
| 5 | | | |
| 6 | | | |
| 7 | | | |
| 8 | | | |
| 9 | | | |
| 10 | | | |

| Development of Motor/Power Skills | | | |
|---|---|---|---|
| **Play** | | | |
| Item | Behaviour | Response | As a result |
| 1 | | | |
| 2 | | | |
| 3 | | | |
| 4 | | | |
| 5 | | | |
| 6 | | | |
| 7 | | | |
| 8 | | | |
| 9 | | | |
| 10 | | | |

| Development of Motor/Power Skills | | | |
|---|---|---|---|
| **Facial Language** | | | |
| Item | Behaviour | Response | As a result |
| 1 | | | |
| 2 | | | |
| 3 | | | |
| 4 | | | |
| 5 | | | |
| 6 | | | |
| 7 | | | |
| 8 | | | |
| 9 | | | |
| 10 | | | |

| Development of Motor/Power Skills | | | |
| Flexibility | | | |
| Item | Behaviour | Response | As a result |
|---|---|---|---|
| 1 | | | |
| 2 | | | |
| 3 | | | |
| 4 | | | |
| 5 | | | |
| 6 | | | |
| 7 | | | |
| 8 | | | |
| 9 | | | |
| 10 | | | |

| Development of Motor/Power Skills | | | |
| Self-care | | | |
| Item | Behaviour | Response | As a result |
|---|---|---|---|
| 1 | | | |
| 2 | | | |
| 3 | | | |
| 4 | | | |
| 5 | | | |
| 6 | | | |
| 7 | | | |
| 8 | | | |
| 9 | | | |
| 10 | | | |

| Development of Motor/Power Skills | | | |
| Emotional Response | | | |
| Item | Behaviour | Response | As a result |
|---|---|---|---|
| 1 | | | |
| 2 | | | |
| 3 | | | |
| 4 | | | |
| 5 | | | |
| 6 | | | |
| 7 | | | |
| 8 | | | |
| 9 | | | |
| 10 | | | |

| Development of Motor/Power Skills | | | |
| --- | --- | --- | --- |
| Get dressed | | | |
| Item | Behaviour | Response | As a result |
| 1 | | | |
| 2 | | | |
| 3 | | | |
| 4 | | | |
| 5 | | | |
| 6 | | | |
| 7 | | | |
| 8 | | | |
| 9 | | | |
| 10 | | | |

| Development of Motor/Power Skills | | | |
| --- | --- | --- | --- |
| Bathroom Use | | | |
| Item | Behaviour | Response | As a result |
| 1 | | | |
| 2 | | | |
| 3 | | | |
| 4 | | | |
| 5 | | | |
| 6 | | | |
| 7 | | | |
| 8 | | | |
| 9 | | | |
| 10 | | | |

| Name: | |
| Age: | Date of birth: |
| Affiliation: | |

**Historical:**

**1. Objectives to be achieved and how to achieve them:**

**2. Tasks (Contents):**

**3. Concrete Materials:**

**4. Resources:**

**5. Considerations / Observations:**

| Primary Skills | | | |
|---|---|---|---|
| | Background | As a result | Response/Content of action |
| | | | |
| | | | |
| | | | |
| | | | |

| Personal Skills (Basic Care/Autonomy) | | | |
|---|---|---|---|
| | Background | As a result | Response/Content of action |
| | | | |
| | | | |
| | | | |
| | | | |

| Playing Skills (Imitation and Repetition) | | | |
|---|---|---|---|
| | Background | As a result | Response/Content of action |
| | | | |
| | | | |
| | | | |
| | | | |

| Expressive Language Skills | | | |
|---|---|---|---|
| | Background | As a result | Response/Content of action |
| | | | |
| | | | |
| | | | |
| | | | |

## Receptive Language Skills

|  | Background | As a result | Response/Content of action |
|---|---|---|---|
|  |  |  |  |
|  |  |  |  |
|  |  |  |  |
|  |  |  |  |

## Social Skills

|  | Background | As a result | Response/Content of action |
|---|---|---|---|
|  |  |  |  |
|  |  |  |  |
|  |  |  |  |
|  |  |  |  |

## Motor Skills

|  | Background | As a result | Response/Content of action |
|---|---|---|---|
|  |  |  |  |
|  |  |  |  |
|  |  |  |  |
|  |  |  |  |

## Augmentative Communication

|  | Background | As a result | Response/Content of action |
|---|---|---|---|
|  |  |  |  |
|  |  |  |  |
|  |  |  |  |
|  |  |  |  |

# PIZZA CURRICULAR

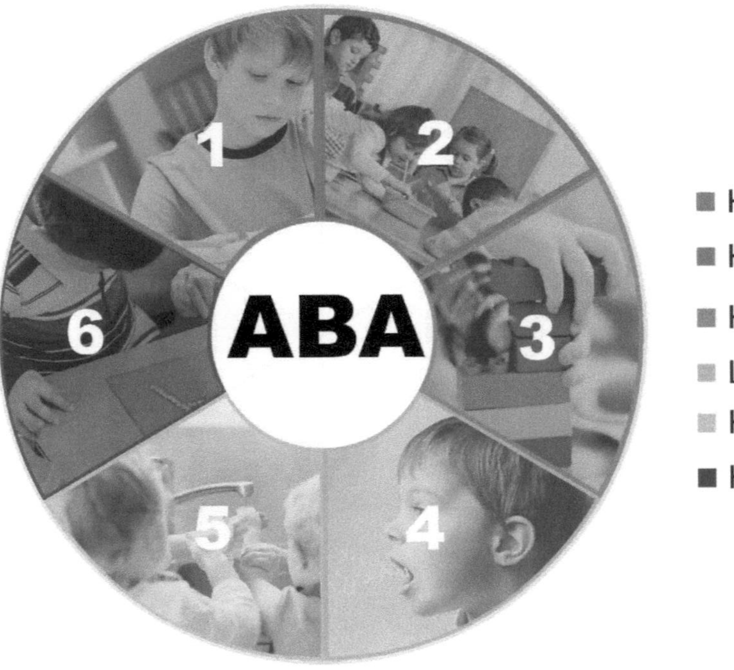

# ACTIVITIES

**Sensory system and sensory integration**

Stereotypes can be replaced by desirable and socially acceptable behaviour. The impairment in the processing of sensory information can lead to hypo or hypersensitivity, which constitutes the B4 diagnostic criteria - hyper or hyporreativity, with symptoms from sensory stimuli or unusual interest in sensory aspects; apparent indifference to pain/temperature, reaction contrary to sounds or textures and visual fascination with light or movement. The fact that it is possible to manage the techniques of sensory integration in multi-modality environments gives this application a practical and extremely functional character. Examples of this type of damage can be tactile (textures, clothes, shoes, etc.), hearing (sound, various sounds and sound effects), visual (images, lights and light effects), gustation (distinction of tastes and avoidance diet), olfaction (distinction of odours and greater or lesser sensitivity to the interpretation of odours).

The activities below enable sensory integration, through PSA/Curriculum, in the development of academic playing skills (HB), by Incidental Teaching or NET. Based on the sensory system, presented in the updated edition of the Atlas of the Human Body, describe the different reactions of our organism when receiving stimuli from the environment.

1. **Fitting sets, legos and puzzles:**

   **Develops skills using the child's psychomotricity and logical reasoning.**

2. **Playing guessing games (using object shapes to identify them). Keeping your eyes closed and walking in a straight line (make sure the space is planned for the activity).**

3. Experience in several different textures (gelatinous, pointed, rough, soft, etc).

4. Wheel and rotate movement and front to back (activities that make it possible to apply laterality, spatiality, gravity).

5. Sensory box, sensory panel and sensory mat (various activities presenting the various possibilities of sensory experiences).

# TARGETED ACTIVITIES

1. **The psychodiagnostic criteria present in the Disorders of Neurological Development (299.00/F84.0) with deficits that are persistent in various contexts are related:**

a)  Social communication and interaction, with motor damage.

b)  Fixity, apraxia and disintegration of childhood skills.

c)  Intellectual compromises in all degrees and motor tics.

d)  Catatonia, compulsion and sensory changes.


2. **On the diagnostic criteria of Autistic Spectrum Disorder, please indicate the corresponding alternative:**

| RECIPROCITY SOCIOEMOTIONAL | BEHAVIOUR COMMUNICATIVE | UNDERSTANDING OF RELATIONSHIPS |
|---|---|---|
| Abnormal social approach | Damage to non-verbal communication | Deficit of adaptation to social contexts |
| Harmful social responses | Variation of verbal and non-verbal communication deficit poorly integrated with abnormality | Damage in sharing imaginary jokes |
| Reduced sharing of interests, emotions or affection | Deficit in understanding facial gestures and expressions | Disinterest in peers and enturmation |
| Diagnostic criteria | Diagnostic criteria | Diagnostic criteria |

Source: Brazilian Association of Psychosomatic Medicine-MT

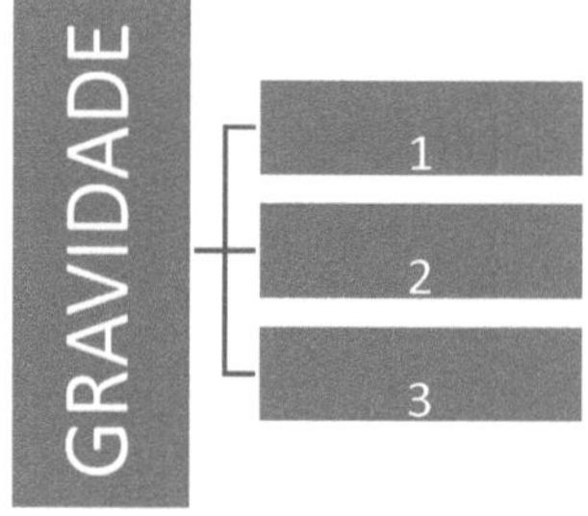


Source: Brazilian Association of Psychosomatic Medicine-MT

a) Criteria A

b) Criteria B

c) Criteria C

d) Criteria D

## 3. On the diagnostic criteria of Autistic Spectrum Disorder, please indicate the corresponding alternative:

| MOVEMENTS ENGINES | INSISTANCE IN MESMICE | INTERESTS FIXES | HIPER OR HYPORREATIVITY |
|---|---|---|---|
| Inappropriate use of objects | Unrelenting adherence to routines | Restricted interests | Sensory stimuli or unusual interest in sensory aspects |
| Stereotyped or repetitive speech, echolalia and idiosyncratic phrases | Ritualized patterns of verbal behaviour | Abnormality and intensity and focus | Apparent indifference to pain/temperature, reaction contrary to sounds or textures |
| Simple motor stereotype, aligning toys or rotating objects | Rigid standards of thought and eating the same food daily | Attachment to unusual objects, circumscribed or persevering interests | Visual fascination by light or movement |
| Diagnostic criteria | Diagnostic criteria | Criteria diagnostics | Criteria diagnostics |

Source: Brazilian Association of Psychosomatic Medicine-MT

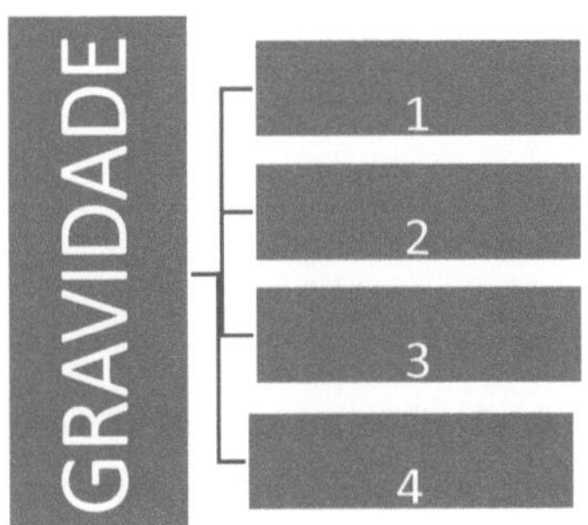


Source: Brazilian Association of Psychosomatic Medicine-MT

a) Criteria A

b) Criteria B

c) Criteria C

d) Criteria D

4. **On the diagnostic criteria of Autistic Spectrum Disorder, please indicate the corresponding alternative:**

| Clinically significant damage to social and professional functioning. |
| --- |
| Diagnostic criteria |

a) Criteria A

b) Criteria B

c) Criteria C

d) Criteria D

5. **On the diagnostic criteria of Autistic Spectrum Disorder, please indicate the corresponding alternative:**

| Specify: with or without concomitant intellectual impairment, with or without concomitant language impairment, with catatonia. |
| --- |
| Diagnostic criteria |

a) Criteria A

b) Criteria C

c) Criteria D

d) Criteria E

6. **Applied Behavior Analysis is an area of knowledge that extends to analysis, explanation, and association with the environment,__spectrum, but with significant potential results in ICD(s) F.84.0 and F.84.1 (Child and Atypical).**

   **The expression that fills the gap in the above text is:**

a) Human behaviour

b) Motor behaviour

c) Verbal behaviour

d) Social behaviour

**7. By centralizing its analysis on the behaviour, it is possible to elaborate a sequential action plan (PSA), in order to act on the behaviour from the behaviourist formula ($^{SD}$ - R# - R/Renforcement +/-). The R# is equivalent:**

a) The different functions in responding to the discriminatory stimulus.

b) To the initial skills development ($^{SD}$) commands.

c) To the tips of answers (modeling, gestural, physical and verbal partial and total).

d) To the verbal operators in the NET curriculum.

**8. The ABA/TEA method as an intervention proposal, mainly in children with signs and symptoms of Autism Spectrum Disorder has in its most significant contribution the elaboration of a curriculum that meets the specific needs of the child's social life and it is in this segment that the ABA/TEA is inserted:**

a) PSA

b) PEI

c) ITP

d) PDI

**9. In the curriculum to be followed there is a sequence of selection, this sequencing being developed by the skills:**

a) Language, social, personal (basic care), play and motor.

b) Individuals, academics, planning and playfulness.

c) Psychomotricity, attitudinal, procedural and conceptual.

d) Relational, motor, intellectual and emotional.

**10.** In an evaluation of the receptive and expressive capacity of language, it is important to evaluate the intrinsic aspects of each instance of reception or expression, even if there are assumptions between them. Mark the alternative that presents a hierarchy in the stimuli of receptive language:

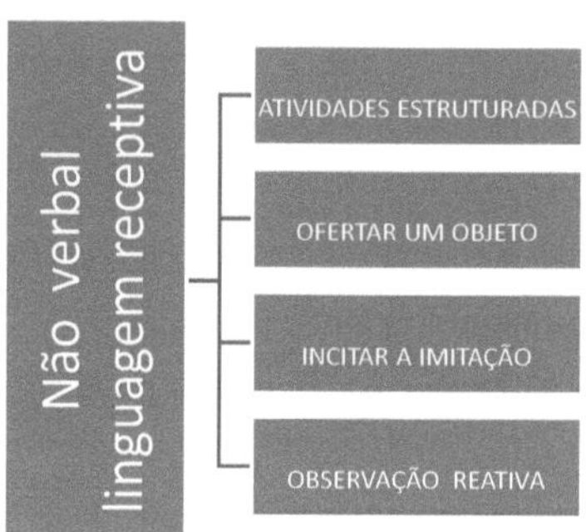


Source: Brazilian Association of Psychosomatic Medicine-MT

a) Structured activities, offering an object, encouraging imitation and reactive observation.

b) Encourage imitation, reactive observation, structured activities and offering an object.

c) Offer an object, encourage imitation, reactive observation and structured activities.

d) Reactive observation, encouraging imitation, structured activities and offering an object.

## LAW NO. 12.764, DECEMBER 27, 2012.

> Establishes the National Policy for the Protection of the Rights of Persons with Autism Spectrum Disorder; and amends § 3 of art. 98 of Law nº 8.112, of December 11, 1990.

**The PRESIDENT OF THE REPUBLIC I hereby** announce that the National Congress decrees and I sanction the following law:

Art. 1 This Law establishes the National Policy for the Protection of the Rights of the Person with Autism Spectrum Disorder and establishes guidelines for its achievement.

§ For the purposes of this Law, a person with autism spectrum disorder is considered to have a clinical syndrome characterized in the form of the following incisors I or II:

I - persistent and clinically significant deficiency of social communication and interaction, manifested by a marked deficiency of verbal and non-verbal communication used for social interaction; absence of social reciprocity; failure to develop and maintain appropriate relationships at their level of development;

II - restrictive and repetitive patterns of behaviour, interests and activities, manifested by motor or verbal stereotyped behaviours or by unusual sensory behaviours; excessive adherence to ritualized routines and patterns of behaviour; restricted and fixed interests.

§ 2 A person with autistic spectrum disorder is considered a person with a disability for all legal purposes.

§ 3 The public and private establishments referred to in Law No. 10,048 of 8 November 2000 may use the jigsaw puzzle ribbon, the global symbol of awareness of autistic spectrum disorder, to identify the priority due to people with autistic spectrum disorder.        (Included by Law No. 13,977 of 2020)

Art. 2 - Guidelines of the National Policy for the Protection of the Rights of Persons with Autism Spectrum Disorder:

I - intersectoriality in the development of actions and policies and in the care of the person with autistic spectrum disorder;

II - community participation in the formulation of public policies aimed at people with autism spectrum disorder and the social control of their implementation, monitoring and evaluation;

III - comprehensive attention to the health needs of the person with autistic spectrum disorder, aiming at early diagnosis, multiprofessional care and access to medicines and nutrients;

IV - (VETADO);

V - the stimulation of the insertion of the person with autism spectrum disorder in the labour market, observing the peculiarities of the disability and the provisions of Law No. 8069 of 13 July 1990 (Statute of the Child and Adolescent);

VI - the responsibility of public authorities for public information concerning the disorder and its implications;

VII - the encouragement of the formation and training of professionals specialized in the care of the person with autistic spectrum disorder, as well as parents and guardians;

VIII - the stimulation of scientific research, with priority for epidemiological studies aimed at dimensioning the magnitude and characteristics of the problem related to the autistic spectrum disorder in the country.

Single paragraph. In order to comply with the guidelines set out in this article, the public authorities may sign a public law contract or an agreement with private law legal entities.

Art. 3 are rights of the person with autistic spectrum disorder:

I - dignified life, physical and moral integrity, free development of personality, security and leisure;

II - protection against any form of abuse and exploitation;

III - access to health actions and services, with a view to comprehensive attention to your health needs, including

a) early, though not definitive, diagnosis;

b) multiprofessional assistance;

c) adequate nutrition and nutritional therapy;

d) medicines;

e) information to assist in diagnosis and treatment;

IV - access:

a) education and vocational education;

b) the dwelling, including the protected residence;

c) the labour market;

d) social security and social assistance.

Single paragraph. In cases of proven necessity, the person with autistic spectrum disorder included in the common classes of regular education, under the terms of item IV of art. 2 , shall be entitled to a specialized escort.

Art. 3a. The Identification Card of the Person with Autism Spectrum Disorder (Ciptea) is created, with a view to guaranteeing integral attention, prompt attendance and priority in the attendance and access to public and private services, especially in the areas of health, education and social assistance. (Included by Law No. 13,977 of 2020)

§ 1º The Ciptea will be issued by the organs responsible for the execution of the National Policy of Protection of the Rights of the Person with Autism Spectrum Disorder of the States, the Federal District and the Cities, by request, accompanied by a medical report, with indication of the code of the International Statistical Classification of Diseases and Problems Related to Health (CID), and must contain, at least, the following information: (Included by Law 13.977, of 2020)

I - full name, affiliation, place and date of birth, civil identity card number, Individual Taxpayer Registration Number (CPF), blood type, full residential address and telephone number of the identified person; (Included by Law No. 13,977 of 2020)

II - photograph in 3 (three) centimetres (cm) x 4 (four) centimetres (cm) format and signature or fingerprint of the identifier; (Included by Law No 13.977 of 2020)

III - full name, identification document, residential address, telephone number and e-mail address of the legal guardian or caregiver; (Included by Law 13.977, of 2020)

IV - identification of the unit of the Federation and of the sending body and signature of the responsible officer. (Included by Law No. 13,977 of 2020)

§ Paragraph 2 In cases where the person with autistic spectrum disorder is an immigrant holding a temporary visa or a residence permit, a border resident or a refugee applicant, the Foreigner Identity Card (CIE), the National Migration Registry Card (CRNM) or the Provisional National Migration Registry Document (DPRNM), valid throughout the national territory, must be presented. (Included by Law no. 13.977, of 2020)

§ 3º Ciptea will be valid for 5 (five) years, and the cadastral data of the identified person must be kept updated, and must be revalidated with the same number, in order to allow the counting of people with autistic spectrum disorder throughout the national territory. (Included by Law no. 13,977 of 2020)

§ 4 Until the provisions in the **caput of** this article are implemented, the bodies responsible for implementing the National Policy for the Protection of the Rights of Persons with Autism Spectrum Disorder shall work together with the respective persons responsible for issuing identification documents, so that the necessary information on autistic spectrum disorder is included in the General Registry (RG) or, if foreigner, in the National Migration Registry Card (CRNM) or the Foreigner Identity Card (CIE), valid throughout the national territory. (Included by Law no. 13.977, of 2020)

Art. 4 The person with autistic spectrum disorder will not be subjected to inhuman or degrading treatment, will not be deprived of his liberty or of family coexistence, nor will he suffer discrimination on the grounds of disability.

Single paragraph. In cases of need for medical hospitalization in specialized units, the provisions of art. 4 of Law nº 10.216, of 6 April 2001, shall be observed.

Art. 5 The person with autistic spectrum disorder will not be prevented from participating in private health care plans due to his or her condition as a disabled person, as provided for in Art. 14 of Law No. 9.656 of 3 June 1998.

Art. 6 (VETADO).

Art. 7 The school manager, or competent authority, who refuses to register a student with autistic spectrum disorder, or any other type of disability, will be punished with a fine from 3 (three) to 20 (twenty) minimum wages.

§ Paragraph 1 In the event of a recidivism, established by administrative procedure, the adversarial procedure and the broad defence shall be ensured, the position shall be lost.

§ 2 (VETADO).

Art. 8 This Law comes into force on the date of its publication.

Brasília, 27 December 2012; 191st of Independence and 124th of the Republic.

DILMA ROUSSEFF
*José Henrique Paim FernandesMiriam Belchior*

<u>**DECREE NO. 8.368, OF 2 DECEMBER 2014**</u>

> Regulates Law No. 12,764 of 27 December 2012, which establishes the National Policy for the Protection of the Rights of Persons with Autism Spectrum Disorder.

**THE PRESIDENT OF THE REPUBLIC,** in the use of the attribution conferred upon her by art. 84, **caput**, item IV, of the Constitution, and in view of the provisions of Law no. 12.764, of December 27, 2012,

**DECREES:**

Art. 1 The person with autistic spectrum disorder is considered a person with disability for all legal purposes.

Single paragraph. The rights and obligations under the International Convention on the Rights of Persons with Disabilities and its Optional Protocol, promulgated by <u>Decree No. 6,949 of 25 August 2009,</u> and the relevant legislation for persons with disabilities, apply to persons with autism spectrum disorder.

Art. 2 The right to health within the Single Health System - SUS is guaranteed to the person with autistic spectrum disorder, respecting their specificities.

§ 1 The Ministry of Health is responsible:

I - to promote the qualification and articulation of the actions and services of the Health Care Network for adequate health care for people with autistic spectrum disorder, to ensure:

a) comprehensive care in the field of basic, specialised and hospital care;

b) the expansion and strengthening of oral health care services for people with an autistic spectrum in basic, specialised and hospital care; and

c) the qualification and strengthening of the psychosocial care network and the health care network for people with autism spectrum disorder, involving differential diagnosis, early stimulation, habilitation, rehabilitation and other procedures defined by the unique therapeutic project;

II - to ensure the availability of drugs incorporated into the SUS necessary for the treatment of people with autistic spectrum disorder;

III - to support and promote processes of permanent education and technical qualification of the professionals of the Health Care Network regarding the care of people with autistic spectrum disorder;

IV - to support research aimed at improving health care and improving the quality of life of people with autistic spectrum disorder; and

V - adopt clinical and therapeutic guidelines with guidelines concerning the health care of people with autism spectrum disorder, observing their specificities of accessibility, communication and care.

§ 2 Health care for the person with autistic spectrum disorder will be based on the International Classification of Functioning, Disability and Health - ICF and the International Classification of Diseases - ICD-10.

Art. 3 Social protection is guaranteed to the person with autistic spectrum disorder in situations of vulnerability or social or personal risk, under the terms of Law nº 8.742, of December 7, 1993.

Art. 4 It is the duty of the State, the family, the school community and society to ensure the right of the person with autism spectrum disorder to education, in an inclusive educational system, by guaranteeing the transversality of special education from early childhood education to higher education.

§ 1 The right addressed in the **caput** shall be ensured in education policies, without discrimination and on the basis of equal opportunities, in accordance with the precepts of the International Convention on the Rights of Persons with Disabilities.

§ 2 If the need for support for communication, social interaction, locomotion, food and personal care activities is proven, the educational institution in which the person with autistic spectrum disorder or other disability is enrolled shall provide specialized accompaniment in the school context, in accordance with the sole paragraph of art. 3 of Law no. 12.764, of 2012.

Article 5 Upon becoming aware of the refusal to register, the competent body shall hear the school manager and decide on the imposition of the fine referred to in the caput of Article 7 of Law No. 12.764 of 2012.

§ Paragraph 1 The Ministry of Education shall be responsible for imposing the fine referred to in the **caput,** in the context of the educational establishments linked to it and of private higher education institutions, in compliance with the procedure provided for in Law No. 9784 of 29 January 1999.

§ 2 The Ministry of Education will inform the Public Prosecutor's Office and the National Council for the Rights of Persons with Disabilities - Conade of the administrative proceedings for imposition of the fine.

§ 3 The amount of the fine shall be calculated on the basis of the number of registrations refused by the manager, the justifications provided and the recidivism.

Art. 6 Any interested party may denounce the refusal of registration of students with disabilities to the competent administrative body.

Art. 7 The public federal body that becomes aware of the refusal to enrol persons with disabilities in educational institutions linked to state, district or municipal education systems shall communicate the refusal to the competent bodies by the respective education systems and to the Public Prosecutor's Office.

Art. 8 The Office of Human Rights of the Presidency of the Republic, together with the Conad, will promote awareness campaigns on the rights of people with autistic spectrum disorder and their families.

Art. 9 This Decree comes into force on the date of its publication.

Brasília, 2 December 2014; 193rd of Independence and 126th of the Republic.

DILMA ROUSSEFF
*José Henrique Paim FernandesArthur*
*ChiorIdeli*
*Salvatti*

# Photographic Records

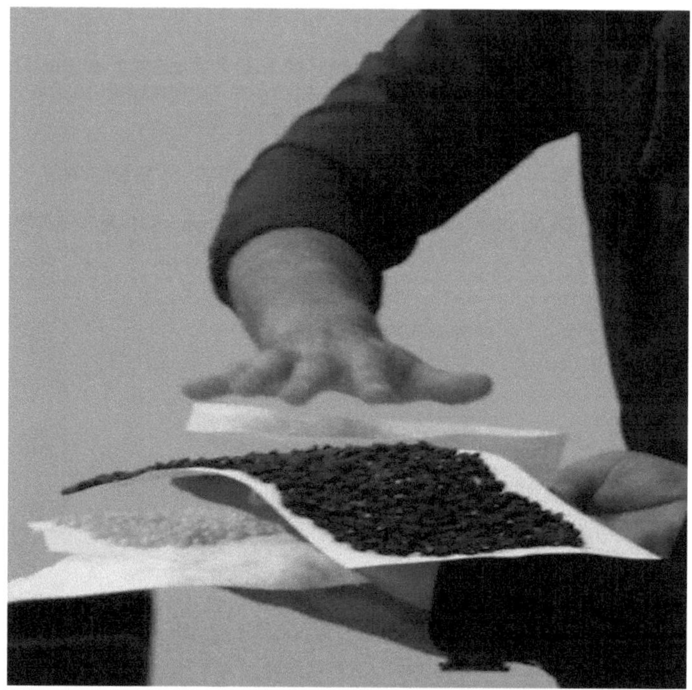

Fig.1 - Evaluation of sensory stimuli: desensitization

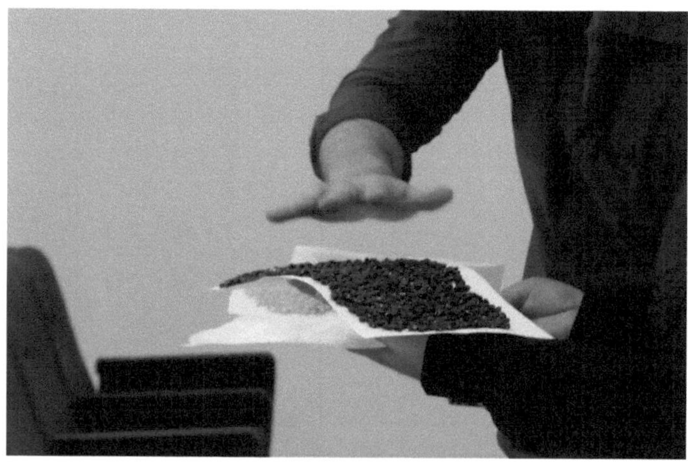

Fig. 2 - Evaluation of sensory stimuli: desensitization

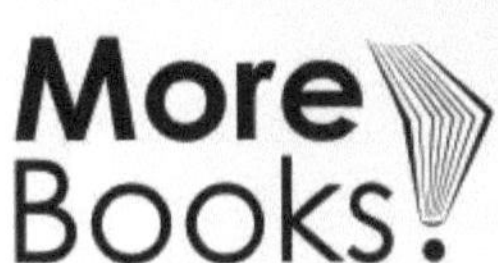

More
Books!


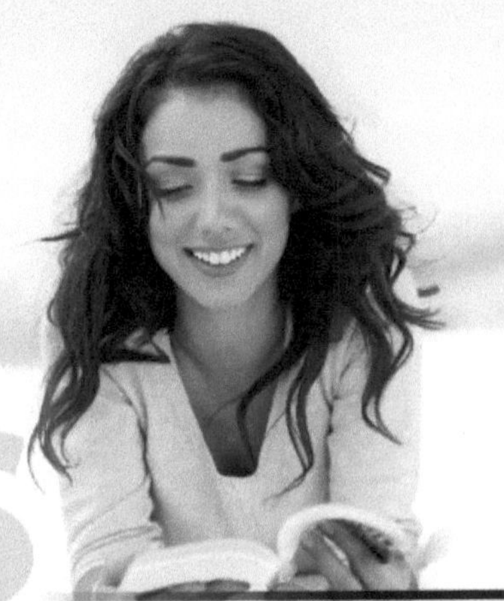



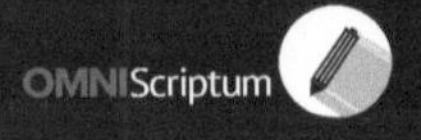

OMNIScriptum

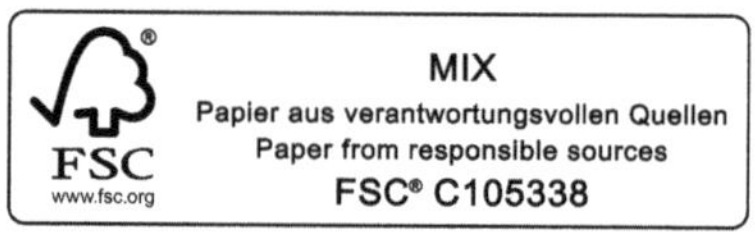


Printed by Books on Demand GmbH, Norderstedt / Germany